HEALTH

beyond

Belief

*Breaking the Beliefs
that block our birthright
for radiant health.*

Doreen Carrie and Pat Comforti

Life Zones Services, Inc.
520 W. 8th Street, Plainfield, New Jersey, 07060
#908-754-5988

The information in this book is for educational purposes only and not intended for diagnosing or prescribing. If the reader uses the information to solve his own health problems, he is prescribing for himself, which is his constitutional right, but the authors and publisher assume no responsibility.

Library of Congress Catalog Card Number 97-072319
ISBN# 0-9650464-0-0
Cover Design: Tom Wood
Text Design: Annette Zindel
Printed in the United States of America

Therefore I say unto you,
what things so ever ye desire,
when ye pray,
believe that ye receive them,
and ye shall have them.

Mark 11:24

Health is no longer the 'exception' to this rule. . .

To
Dr. Thurman Fleet,
founder of the
Concept-Therapy Institute,
who helped to build
the bridge of health that
others may cross.
Dr. Fleet prophesied that
the day would come
when radiant health and
fully functional living
would be realized
by all human souls.
With eternal gratitude and love
we dedicate this book,
hoping to further
his magnificent prophecy.

CONTENTS

Acknowledgments

This book could never have been written without the total love and support of our husbands. Living with us during this two year project hasn't been easy on them. They have had to be patient, encouraging, trusting and extra loving to two sometimes very frazzled women with a mission who didn't always have dinner ready on time or remember the cleaning.

So many extra miles walked, so much uplifting encouragement when we needed it most. When we worked til midnight, when we needed a proof reader, when we just needed our space, they took the children without a question or made us a cup of tea. To Don and Allen, with all our love and appreciation for truly being the extraordinary men in our lives.

To our children Caitlin Rose and Jaclyn Taylor, who have taught us more about our true selves and true healing than we would ever have learned on our own in a lifetime. You make us smile and warm our hearts when we need it most with just a hug.

To Annette Zindel and Tom Wood who have gone well beyond the call of duty and friendship for all the hours of time put in on your own, our heartfelt thanks.

To our parents, Al, Marian, Stella and Stan for giving us the strength, confidence and guidance to know that we could succeed at anything we put our hearts into. Your support was unconditional as we pursued a career and life path that at times seemed destined for failure.

We owe this book and our sanity to all of you.

Introduction to Healing our Sick Approach to Health

We live in an age where the quality of life has never been better. Never before has there been more life enhancing progress, more realization of our God given unlimitedness or more hope for the future. Unfortunately, *health* is the exception to this rule.

After twelve years of research - with people, not animals - this book dares to question and disagree with today's system of health; a system that accepts headaches, backaches, colds, the flu, allergies, fatigue and chronic health problems as a normal part of life. Normal, yes, but *natural*. . . far from it. Our natural state - ease, energy and exuberance - has been squelched in a system that fills our minds with everything that *could* go wrong with the body. We have been led to believe that focusing on the warning signs and vivid pictures of *sickness* will somehow bring us *health*. 'B.S.'!

Inner 'B.S.' - Belief Systems - create our outer life. We accept this principle for our careers, relationships and for every goal we desire. Why then, has health become the tragic exception to this rule? Have we forgotten that the very essence of our being is unlimited creative spirit, granting us the ability to create the life and the *health* that we want? Maybe we haven't forgotten, maybe we have never been told. Fueled by the multi-billion dollar medical and advertising field, the 'sick' approach that society has taken with health - focusing on and fearing illness - has kept us in ignorance of our unlimited healing power within. What's more, we have been led to believe that *not being sick* is the best we can hope for with health. Is there no end to the 'B.S.'?

We are governed by a health system that puts all its energy into preventing and curing sickness. Aside from the obvious fact that this approach has some major bugs in it - even after billions of dollars spent in research, pain, fatigue and illness are at an all time high -

this system passes right over a special but forgotten group. What about the majority of us who are *well*, relatively speaking? Should we conclude that our potential for health has been tapped just because we are *not sick*? Not unless we would conclude that our potential for success has been tapped just because we are *not failing*. A principle that applies to one area of life applies to all, no exception. There is a *whole* other side of health just waiting for those who *are not sick but far from radiant*. Rich, vibrant health - ease, energy and a feeling of exuberance - is the next step in our potential for health. What doctor, hospital or insurance carrier, however, is able to lead us to this exuberant state? Our Health Care System as it now stands, is set up to treat the *sick*. But for those of us who want to get off the 'sick to not sick' merry-go-round and on to our right to radiance, the system does not work!

This book addresses our right, our divine birthright, for radiance. First, it helps us get beyond the 'B.S.' that has kept us bound to our chronic aches, pains, fatigues and ills; suffering is not part of the Divine Plan. Then it leads us to a whole new level of health, well beyond ground '0', which is the absence of symptoms. The '0'-100% realm, our natural state, but far above the norm, is the beginning of bliss, the real goal of health. This book introduces us to our unlimited power within, a power that heals not only a body but a life.

Although the world is literally dying for this unlimited approach to health, not everyone is dying to do what it takes. A person who is satisfied with their present state of health and believes that they are adequately 'insured' for the future is not a candidate for "**Health beyond *Belief*.**" This higher state of health requires taking on a true degree of responsibility for health, well beyond cutting cholesterol, exercising or abstaining from nicotine. Healing the negative beliefs in our mind and opening up to the unlimited creative power within, are our real responsibilities and the ultimate purpose of this book.

"Health beyond *Belief*" bridges a much needed gap; the gap between the spiritual and the physical; between our spiritual unlimitedness and our physical life. For too long we have been *told* about our God given right to create the life that we want, but the *how to do it* has until now, been virtually ignored.

Bottomline, there is nothing that stands between us and our birthright for an abundant, fully potentialized life, nothing except our own 'B.S.' And with this book, *health* is no longer the exception to that rule.

Preface

There is a story in everyone's life, a reason that the events of our life unfold as they do. If you have taken on the task of self actualization, you know there is a divine purpose for your life. You have come to trust in a power that always leads you to your highest good. If, however, you have not yet taken on this task, but have a sense that there is more to life - a better way - you've come to the right place.

From this point on, as the events in your own personal 'book of life,' reveal their meaning, you can, with awareness, be led to your Divine destiny. In this book we share our personal story and the truths that we have learned in the hope of helping you open to this divine destiny; radiant health being one of its rewards. That is the purpose of **Health Beyond** *Belief.*

Rebels *with* a Cause

If you had told Pat & Doreen when they first became business part-
ners that it was their mission to help revolutionize the health industry and to dedicate their lives to physical, mental and spiritual
health, they would have said "You're joking, right?"

Doreen's Story:

Health and Fitness was the last thing that I or anyone else expected
to be my career. In 1980 I graduated from Rutger's University with
a degree in Business and Accounting, a far cry from health. I even
connived my way out of college gym class every year due to 'health'
reasons. Neither coordination nor team sports were my strong
points. So how did I come years later to create a great exercise
program and ultimately a highly effective wholistic health system,
when my degree said I was a qualified accountant? Well, degrees
can be misleading. After a disastrous year working for one of the
world's largest 'health' conglomerates (health was really their front
for selling pharmaceuticals), I wondered how I ever graduated.

I should have gotten the message that I had no head for accounting.
Totally confused and scared to death of failing, I bought the answers to the final exams. You'd think with the answers in my
grubby little hands that I would have aced the exam. Well think
again! I soon learned that if the concept was beyond a person, even
having the answers can't help. I got a 'D' by the skin of my teeth,
and if it weren't for course electives like drama, public speaking, abnormal psychology and human sexuality, (my real talents), I would
have failed out of college.

My 'degree' said that I was an accountant but it was just a matter of
time until my less than adequate skills began to surface. Ironically I
landed a great accounting job right out of college, but the first day
on the job foretold my future. My boss asked me to do a rather

elementary task for a graduate accountant, to add a group of numbers for a meeting with his V.P. The look on his face after the meeting told me that I might have made a slight mathematical error. I had misplaced the decimal point so instead of the correct total of $5,000,000, I left my boss with the humiliating job of explaining how he had come up with $50,000. It was right then and there that I knew my accounting days were numbered. That, followed by a few more disasters quickly ended my calamity as an accountant; a venture I had no business taking on.

Looking back, I can now see the creative writing on the walls. Rather than relying on my four year college degree to decide my talents - as so many creative people unfortunately do - if I had looked at my drives and loves over the years, I would have clearly seen my path.

Almost before I could talk, I was drawing, painting, sculpting, and finding more ingenious ways to enjoy childhood. I cannot remember ever being bored, although it was a daily complaint for most of my friends. Boredom was never my problem; incessant creativity and a bedroom that resembled an art explosion was. Why didn't I see back then that my talent was not exactly accounting oriented? More to the point, why hadn't my high school guidance counselors seen that I use my boundless creativity instead of banging my head against the wall with accounting? Well, whatever the reason, it was now 1981 and I was out of a job and a career within a year of graduation. Oddly though instead of feeling like a failure, for the first time in years I felt free. Completely turned off by the corporate climate, I supplemented my income with a variety of odd jobs; some odder than others. Imagine my parents reaction when they heard that their college graduate was now painting signs on delivery trucks! And they still supported me, thank God. The odd jobs ended quickly but I remained without a clear direction. Somehow I knew that if I couldn't find my path, it would just have to find me.

One day while exercising at my health spa, (my least favorite activity ironically), a member, trying to create an exercise business of her own, asked me if I ever thought about teaching aerobics. I lied and said, "yes, all the time!" On that she invited me to practice sessions in her basement. Just being happy someone wanted me for something, I neglected the fact that I was totally uncoordinated and not good at following directions. I tripped over my own feet and messed up some of the other trainees, but I was determined. Unfortunately, the woman who had created this business was having her own problems. Every time I would call her about an organization that wanted her aerobic classes she would be sick in bed with a migraine. She promised to call me back but she never did. Almost ready to give up, it dawned on me; why not create my own aerobic classes? Never doubting my ability - although I had about as much training in aerobics as nuclear physics - I convinced everyone who later registered for my classes that I was an expert.

Before I knew it newspapers were running stories on my classes and people were lining up to get in! This proved that the spiritual asset of *creative genius* which everyone has, is far more powerful than academic knowledge or IQ. My classes were created to build up a person's self esteem, allowing each person to express themselves freely and sensually. These classes were less about 'exercise' and more about 'self expression,' a quality desperately needed in our stiff society.

In less than a year I went from a failed accountant to creating a flourishing business; creating being the operative word. Almost overnight I had more classes than I could handle and was bringing in a great income. I finally felt right with my direction. I loved teaching and creating aerobics; my classes were filled to capacity and new ones were ready to be set up. So how come I felt that something was missing? Even though I loved to create and could spend hours alone thinking of new ideas, I desperately needed someone with whom to share my dreams and visions; someone who had the same inner calling and would see this mission through to the end.

Pat still says that the first time we talked on the phone I was giving her a sales pitch, but that was not true. I knew from our first conversation that she was the one.

Pat's Story:

An actress, a ruler of a small country or a nun were some of my early career choices. I had been a high honors student since first grade, had a remarkable "IQ" and loved school. So I never understood why I ended up failing out of college.

But at 19, being a creative hippy of the times who loved to philosophize and talk about peace on earth and saving the world, geology, advanced spanish and western civ. bored me to death. The whole atmosphere of college (so big, I had graduated from a small private Catholic girls academy very popular and secure) made me feel unloved, lost and unhappy. All my friends had gone off to other places and I truly felt like a misfit.

The only good friend I made felt just like me (of course) and both of us, bright, enthusiastic and curious would take off days at a time and haunt coffee houses to talk, raid old bookstores and reveal our dreams to each other. This was 1970. My dad had already made me very aware of Concept-Therapy, a philosophy which had changed his life and was about to become the foundation on which I would build mine. My journey led me through a 10 year first marriage, a number of colorful jobs as secretary, waitress, dancer and salesperson. Yet the constant thread that ran through my life was studying, learning, trying to get clear on the idea of God, and my connection to it all.

Concept-Therapy began to play a major part in my life as I took class after class for many years. By 1983, I was qualified to take a

Teacher's Training Course at the Concept-Therapy Headquarters in San Antonio, Texas. I felt very willing to move on to this challenging step. I had just gotten married to my 'perfect mate' and moved to a new home where I saw Doreen's ad for exercise classes.

Doreen and I came from very different backgrounds but we shared a common problem and a common purpose. Both of us considered ourselves *mainstream misfits*. We just couldn't and wouldn't fit into the 'normal,' 9 - 5' corporate world. We also felt strongly that vital areas of life, such as education, women's career paths and health, were in desperate need of an overhaul. We both believed that these three areas were based on backwards, artificial and self suppressing standards. Rather than resign to them, we decided instead to *redesign* them. Our creative, passionate and rather *rebellious* natures matched up perfectly.

1984 began our partnership, a partnership that would teach us the true meaning of friendship and dedication. It would take us many years before we would know our real purpose in this business. In the early days our main goal was to be a huge success in the aerobic field. But we took a detour midstream. Instead of spending the majority of our brainstorming sessions creating ways to take the fitness field by storm, we kept being led to ideas of holistic healing and self realization. Both of us fervently agreed that our society's concept of health and success were backwards and self-destructive. Innately we knew that illness, stress and suffering, even though accepted as a 'normal' part of life, were not the way human beings were intended to live. We also knew that eliminating cholesterol, nicotine and sunbathing were not the solutions to our problems. The cure for our problems and the fulfillment of our desires could not be found in the physical alone.

We had begun to understand that human beings were multidimensional, even though our current health, education and corporate systems were treating us like physical machines, addressing our physical needs only. What about our emotional and spiritual needs?

We certainly had more than one 'zone' to our being. It was about this time that we created the name LIFE ZONES for our business, exemplifying the many zones of our being that needed to be healed, satisfied and potentialized. Primitively we created a program that introduced our unlimited power within. This concept was quite different than the *cure-alls* of the early '80's; nutrition, fitness and a dab of stress management.

During the '80's, we watched the fitness fad peak and crash in less than 10 years. Health clubs owned by casinos and other conglomerates promised to bring us health and happiness for life. Half of Hollywood's stars were making fitness videos, all short-lived. For a reason still unknown to us we had a real mission to create and provide our society with a true 'whole'-istic approach to health. Every avenue of our business from that point on, acted as a *front* for us to discover what that new approach would be.

With a captive audience of hundreds of unsuspecting participants in our aerobic exercise classes, we began experimenting. Our classes were already highly motivational, but now we would elevate them to inspirational. Our classes turned out to be a true *mind/body* experience. We choreographed exercise routines that allowed for free, sensual expression of the body, so our whole being - mind, body and inner self - could flow naturally. A guided meditation to get in touch with our healing energy ended the class. Headaches, stiff necks, back problems, allergies, sinus blockages started either decreasing or disappearing for many of the participants. Ills that had been labeled *chronic* by doctors were lessening. These *mini-healings* surprised the participants, but it proved what we had suspected all along; when a person is really free to be themselves and flow with their true inner nature, (even in exercise) everything in their life, health no exception, is elevated.

We realized in a short time that our aerobic classes gave us the forum to explore and practice the bigger picture of healing that we had begun to understand. Contrary to our fitness colleagues of the time, we knew that self doubt and chronic illnesses could not be healed by aerobics, nonsmoking or cutting all fat from out diets. Healing was an *inside job*. Even though the medical system still tries to convince us that pills, surgery or other physical remedies are the answer, we were seeing something far different in our classes. As participants began looking inside and do some healing of their negative self images, changes occurred. From that moment on, we knew a drug, no matter how 'revolutionary' could never match these results.

Even after a few years we were just scratching the surface of this inner sense. We still tried to force our own lives from the outside, leaving us often frustrated, stressed and sick, but even the tiny bit of this higher self awareness radiated like heat. Much later we realized that the reason so many people flocked to our exercise classes was because they too felt in touch with this higher awareness within them. They were uplifted spiritually even though they were just exercising physically.

When we first met, I was quite involved in Concept-Therapy. I tried to explain to Doreen how this teaching had answered many of my unanswered questions on health, true happiness and God. Like most self doubting, fear run people, Doreen felt life was just fine the way it was. Constant headaches, worry, insecurity, guilt laced with spurts of excitement were normal, right? Resistant and a bit suspicious, she conceded to 'try' the Concept-Therapy class. God knows, though she could not see it then, Doreen's life was in need of a stronger philosophy. Her Jewish religion had done little to ease the pressure of life. Half of the religious services were in Hebrew and how it pertained to her health, relationships and self image problems was a mystery.

Dr. Fleet, the originator of Concept-Therapy in 1931, did all the hard work. He compiled the truths of healing, religion, happiness and self growth; all its participants had to do was study and practice. The thousands of Concept-Therapy participants owe so much, their life in many cases, to Dr. Fleet. Personally we know that *our* life and *our* ability to help others find their higher selves is due to this teaching. To this day Concept-Therapy remains the foundation of our lives and our business.

Like every great philosophy since time began, Concept-Therapy teaches that our divine heritage entitles every person to an unlimited, blissful life. In fact, our *natural* state is one of inner peace, abundance and joy; radiant health being no exception. Then how in the world we wondered, had stress and suffering become the *norm;* rampant illness being no exception? That question gnawed at us day in and day out. If it were so natural to flow with radiance, health being a given, then something had to be blocking this flow.

The Road to Health. . . the Beginning

As far as we could see, no one was really addressing the blocks to the flow of radiant health; the medical establishment surely wasn't. They didn't and still don't acknowledge the fact that radiant health is the natural state. On the contrary, they focus on warning the public of the growing number of illnesses that could strike them. Not all health professionals however, were advocating this rather sick approach to health. Many, especially those involved in alternative practices were proclaiming our right to create the life we want, health being no exception. Thank God for their words of wisdom, but words, even the most inspirational, were only half the picture. Enough people were informing the world about the unlimited life and health that we *could have.* Completing the picture, it became our mission to find out why we *didn't.*

Once we accepted the task of finding out why we *didn't* have the great flow of healing that we *could* and *should,* our eyes and ears became extremely sensitive to the sick view that society had with health. We saw how deeply dyed this consciousness of sickness, stress and self doubt was in the hearts and minds of everyone we met. Our clients, friends and families all complained of some body or life pain. Wherever we were, in a bank, supermarket, restaurant, even a 'health' club, the buzzing of illness invaded our senses. Whether it was the person's own illness or that of their loved one, the endless description of deteriorating body parts became the central theme of conversation with the media backing up these sick conversations. True to our nature and our mission, the more we saw how much society feared and focused on illness, the more determined we became. Our search for the blocks to the flow of natural healing turned from passion to obsession. We listened intently to friends, family members, clients, strangers on the street, (and especially ourselves), looking for clues to these blocks. Maybe it was a special insight, or maybe it was just morbid curiosity, but in many cases we were able to see the connection between a person and their health problems; between a person's thoughts, expectations, self acceptance, spiritual grounding and their particular problem. In the beginning our insights were more jumbled theories than practical solutions, but it definitely felt like we were on the right track.

There was, unfortunately, a down side to our new direction. As a business we had a great mission, but financially speaking we were not looking too solid. Any income we did earn paid the overhead; rent, secretary, phone and other miscellaneous business expenses. As we switched from a successful aerobic business to become researchers to finding the blocks to healing, our income plummeted. We were forced to move out of our beautiful office, let go of our secretary and rent a small, cheaper space on top of a pizza parlour.

The next two years were filled with much frustration and self doubt, often it felt like the weight of the world was on our shoulders. It was hard not to think we were failing especially when our accountant informed us, that from a business point, we were headed down the tubes. Fortunately our mission to find the blocks to healing overshadowed the apparent financial circumstances. Few people around us at the time could understand why we stayed with something that obviously wasn't working while not continuing to stay with selling more of our exercise programs which were working so well. We were often asked by well meaning souls, "Why don't you get a *real* job?" If we were only trying to get a 'job,' or become a financial success, we would probably be selling Tupperware by now. But something inside of us had changed; we had gotten a glimpse into the truth of healing as well as a rather clear view of the sick holes in our current health system. This new consciousness filled our hearts and our souls so powerfully that we had no choice but to follow it through to the end.

We knew that we had taken on quite a worthy task. We also knew even then that it would be a long and arduous one. In the meantime we had to find a way to earn some income. Far from ready to share our new health insights with the world, we saw an opportunity to heal another system, one that we had seen a hole in for a long time. Even though our own traditional education more or less ignored our creative potential, from a nontraditional perspective we knew that we were really geniuses. (Actually every human being is a genius once they connect with their talent). As geniuses, however, we never claim creation of the principles themselves; they have been around and promulgated since time began. Our talent is discovering in what systems these principles have been lost and then creating an exciting and practical way to restore them to usability in everyday life. This is definitely not a talent for which one could get a traditional 'Degree,' but then who said any of us are limited to traditional degrees? And with that idea of a nontraditional approach to education and formal degrees, we were in business again.

It was perfect. Before tackling the auspicious health system, a system revered as another 'God,' we decided to revamp something a little less threatening. For a long time we had seen the hole in traditional education and the need for another kind of 'degree.' In the past few decades, traditional education had certainly advanced, but unfortunately only in one direction. Focused entirely on the *external* - getting a good job, being intellectually learned - traditional education entirely misses the *internal*. Principles like the mind/body connection, ideals like self esteem and self actualization, even spiritual beliefs, (not to be confused with *religious* beliefs), while the very foundation of our lives, are barely if ever discussed in schools today.

In keeping with our rather nontraditional, sometimes rebellious way of doing things - formal education and degrees not required for starting a career path or a whole new system of life for that matter - we set out to heal the holes in traditional education. (Of course we continued with 30 - 45 hours per month of our own education through Concept-Therapy, which unlike traditional education doesn't end after the final exams). From the realization that traditional education focuses entirely on the external, we created what we called an *Internal* Education. We named this internal education, the "DEGREES OF LIFE." Our first of many 'degrees' was the **MBA** or **M**ind **B**ody **A**wakening®. We explained this idea as similar to the traditional degree, only instead of being a graduate degree in *business*, it would be a graduate degree in *life*. The purpose of the **MBA** was to introduce the principles of the mind/body connection and self actualization. It also promoted the rarely discussed fact that true education, derived from its original definition, means to *draw out* what is already within a person. Primarily concerned with *stuffing in* more and more information, traditional education rarely draws out the individual genius, let alone the universal power, within all of us.

While it may have appeared that we were going away from our original mission in health, this was not true at all. The missing 'self' subjects, and the consequent underdevelopment of our self worth, are directly responsible for many of our ills today, (which will be discussed further throughout this book), we were still on the health track, just not quite ready to publicize it as such.

We spent an entire summer putting together the **MBA**. This new project, coupled with our continued research of the healing blocks kept us quite busy. Within a few short but intense months we were ready to present our program. We offered the MBA to over a dozen Adult Schools and they loved it! This was the latter part of the '80's and society was ready to look *inside* for some answers to their *outside* problems since working externally was not producing any lasting results. Our **MBA** students, twenty to thirty in a class, came from all walks of life and all 'degrees' of academic education. None of the external standards to which we normally measure a person's worth mattered here; all quickly learned that when it came to this internal progress, we were all beginners.

Watching this **Mind Body Awakening**® program make some great inner and outer strides with our students, deepened our conviction and confidence of the mind/body principle. Hundreds of people were seeing emotional, physical and spiritual changes in themselves for the first time in their lives, even for some after years of therapy. Once again, however, there was a down side to our achievement. Even an entire semester at an Adult School, eight weeks in most cases, was not nearly long enough to sustain the positive changes. It had taken an entire lifetime to create the conditions that we were trying to heal; it was a long shot to believe a few short months could permanently heal them. We always suggested that the students attend a Concept-Therapy class upon completion of the course, but given the newness of the whole holistic living idea, this was often a long shot for the majority of them, although there were those who did attend and are actively involved with Concept-Therapy today. As for the rest, however, we felt like we were abandoning them just as they were beginning to bring this healing idea into their lives. From that experience we knew that this internal education needed a few years not just a few months to become incorporated into a person's life.

In the hopes of working with a group of people for a year or more, we chose large corporations as our next venture. We also hoped to strike it big financially with this new market. But the immediate acceptance that we found with the Adult School population was far from the same with Corporate America. We definitely needed this experience for our growth but at the time it almost killed our newly healed spirits. Our first mistake was naively believing that corporations were dying for a program like ours; they were dying all right, but they did not see us or our program as the saviors. The second mistake was looking at these big corporations as our financial future. In years to come we would understand a hard but vital lesson; anytime we had 'dollar signs in our eyes,' we would end up with little more than pain in our hearts. At the beginning of our rendezvous with Corporate America, however, that lesson had yet to be learned.

Doesn't anybody want us?

Most of the corporate directors with whom we spoke were actually very open to this new idea of self growth for their employees. The majority of their employees were stressed out, often sick and rarely enthusiastic about their jobs. On top of all that, health care costs were eating up company profits. It seemed therefore, that a program that taught people how to create self esteem, inner calmness and greater health would be a perfect match; the executives were well aware of the employee problems running rampant in their company. Unfortunately being *aware* of the problem was one thing. *Spending money* on an intangible, yet to be proven idea was another. Instead, many health minded corporations at that time figured a couple of yearly blood pressure and cholesterol screenings, some lectures on nutrition, a smoking cessation course and some pamphlets describing the warning signs of heart disease satisfied the company's 'wellness' requirements. As long as it took no time away from business hours and more importantly was inexpensive or free, company executives would be happy to provide the service. Most companies said they were 'people oriented,' (caring about the welfare of their employees), but when push came to shove, spending money on their employees wellness was not a priority.
(Interestingly, they managed to always have enough money for a lavish Christmas party. . .)

We laugh now looking back at ourselves during our corporate experience. Fortunately we were so dedicated to our mission that we failed to see the absurdity of what we were trying to do. Here we were two energetic, passionate women, trying to sell an intangible product to a very bottom line environment; an environment whose main goal was slicing budgets and down sizing personnel. On top of that, we had no real data to support our claims. We quickly found out that just because *we* were sold on our idea didn't mean everyone else would buy it. How could we convince such 'prove it to me' kind of people to invest time and money in a yet to be proven idea? We couldn't. It was one rejection after another. Most of the time the company executives refused to take our calls, human resource directors, ironically being the least interested or perhaps the most frustrated. Many of the interviews that we did get were with assistants who couldn't approve buying more paper towels, much less a wellness program. We were banging our heads on a door that wouldn't open.

We didn't know it then, especially amid the daily fear of losing our business and our self worth, but the door that closed to Corporate America opened our way to making one of the most vital decisions of our career. It was the winter of 1990. We were just about at the breaking point. Professionally we *looked* like a failure and personally we *felt* like one. Yet every day we had to get on the phone with corporations that would have responded better if we were selling water coolers instead of wellness programs. To say that we were not having fun would have been an understatement. On top of that, we were in an old office building that had a temperamental heating system. Talk about 'cold calls!' One day after making our quota of calls dressed in winter coats and gloves, we looked at each other with a determined strength in our eyes and simultaneously said, "That's it." It took less than a day to inform our understanding landlord, move out of our office and vow never again to follow the path of most resistance. We promised each other and Pat's unborn child, (she was five months pregnant at the time), that even if we never made another dime, we would do only those things that gave us joy and purpose. If we had to fail, (in the the business world), we were going to have a blast at it.

Purpose vs. Pocketbook

Without an office and once again without a traditional business, we felt happier and freer than we had in years. Just the thought of never having to make another cold call gave us new joy. Our 'home office' became an office in each of our homes. We continued to meet every day with diners in New Jersey becoming our place of business. To this day we still do our best work over coffee and a salad bar.

It was March of 1990, and without any overhead hanging over our heads, we could choose the path that would best suit our purpose and our passion. We still worked diligently to discover the blocks to healing and we also had a **Mind Body Awakening**® program that gave life to the too often prattled about and too little practiced, 'mind/body connection.' While the thought of making another cold call to a corporation sent shivers down our spine, we needed this environment as much as they needed us. The answers to the blocks to healing as well as helping people awaken to their mind/body connection, our current purpose, could only be accomplished by working with a group of people for at least a year. And as much as we did not like to admit it, Corporate America was the place to do it.

We still, however kept to our promise of only doing things that were both pleasant and productive, cold calls satisfying neither. No longer having the need to prove ourselves, and no attachment to the outcome, (or 'income'), we went for broke. We visualized a corporation first of all calling *us,* then allowing us *carte blanche* with our programs and finally contracting with us for a *minimum of one year.* Also, because of financial strains that both of us were going through at the time, we promised our spouses that we would once again have great salaries by June 1st, only a few months away.

We still shake our heads in awe when we look at the *date* on which we signed our first major corporate contract; June 1st 1990. Herman's World of Sporting Goods was going through a major reorganization, not to mention many layoffs when they contracted with LIFE ZONES, Inc. (us). Since we never doubted our goal, neither did they. Herman's called *us,* gave us *carte blanche* and contracted with us for *one year* with a one year option, our exact goal. It would prove to be a most growing experience, not just for the employees, but for us.

Just landing the Herman's contract in the first place proved once again to us the power of belief over circumstances. Logically we should never have even been considered for the position. We had no previous corporate experience and few references to whom we weren't related. Our credentials - a failed accountant and an ex dancer - were not exactly supporting our health and personal growth claims. To top it off, we were two virtually inexperienced women being hired for a position normally run by accredited health professionals, into a company whose upper management consisted of 99% men.

We still don't think that Herman's management knew what they were in for in the beginning. Originally hired to manage their newly built fitness center, we did that and a 'whole' lot more. Our goal was to provide a whole-istic health service, although advertising it as such was held in abeyance until Herman's got to know us a little better. Rather than ruffling too many feathers by labeling our service a 'health' program, (run by two women with not even a *formal fitness* background), we took the safe approach. We created a LIFE ENRICHMENT Service; it was still more acceptable for a 'non professional' to enrich life than health. Either way, this service was far too much for us to handle alone, especially since Pat had only a month before given birth to her first child. But where would we find someone who was dedicated to true whole-istic health, (far beyond exercise and good nutrition), who would put up with our constant changing and creating, who could handle the monumental task of running a LIFE ENRICHMENT Service?

Jennifer McCarthy, a truly inspired woman, had been hired by Life Zones a year before to teach one of our aerobic classes. Unfortunately the students were not too thrilled with her style of teaching. We fired her from teaching aerobics and hired her to do some clerical work for us. But she couldn't type and her spelling was even worse. What could we do with her? We knew that Jen had something very special to offer, we just hadn't yet figured out what it was. But when we needed someone to create and run this new LIFE ENRICHMENT Service, we had no doubt that Jen could do it. Jen suffered from the same ailment to which many, ourselves included, were afflicted; misdiagnosis of talent and misdirection of career. She had an extraordinary spirit that would not fit into ordinary channels. She also had an openness to true whole-istic living as well as unlimited creativity; two job requirements in our line of work. We knew that she would go above and beyond the call of duty. We were right.

Ironically it was Jen, while tending bar, who made the initial contact for Herman's. We struggled for years to do formal presentations with corporations and Jen clinches a major deal over cocktails! She never expected so much as a finder's fee for connecting us with Herman's, and we are eternally grateful to Jen for her faith in us. It was our mutual faith in each other that made the whole service fly.

This 12 hour a day, 5 day a week LIFE ENRICHMENT Service could not run with Jen alone. Ralph Lardieri and Janice Kluxen, because of their belief in fitness of the self as well as of the body, took the service to new heights. These two had an intense background in physical fitness as well as traditional college degrees, but we didn't hold that against them! Actually their physical fitness knowledge was very helpful as long as they realized that the physical was only a part of the whole picture of health. Too much emphasis on the physical - the 'right' way to exercise, perfect nutrition, checking cholesterol - at the expense of the emotional and spiritual was really an unhealthy way to live. Raising a person's spirit, and educating them on the unlimited healing power within us all, the main purpose of the LIFE ENRICHMENT Service, did more to restore the sparkle in their eyes and the hope in their heart, (true indicators of health), than all the low fat foods and cardiovascular exercises put together. In a short time LIFE ENRICHMENT became a full department in Herman's and a household name. Many times we had heard that employees looking to other companies for employment were shocked that they didn't have a LIFE ENRICH-MENT Service! Herman's even used this service to entice people to work for them. No one had the slightest idea that this whole service was a product of our imagination, created weeks after we were hired. But because of the deep faith we had in the service and its purpose everyone accepted it as though it had been endorsed by Oprah.

We, along with Jen, Ralph and Janice, became a strong team at Herman's. Our philosophies, although quite different in the beginning, became uniformly one within a few months. To this day, we all attend Concept-Therapy classes regularly and are as close in vibration as we were at Herman's. Jen, Ralph and Janice each gave a thousand percent, doing their job so well that we were free to do ours.

Exercise was important, but education was our real purpose. Workshops became the forum from which to introduce a much needed internal education. Our first workshop, the **Mind Body Awakening**® was received quite well. It was basically an easy to understand, nonthreatening introduction to self worth and the mind/body connection; these two subjects had recently received society's stamp of approval, so we faced little resistance with the employees. Perhaps it was because of the way we inspired people or maybe it was the fact that employees were allowed to attend the workshops on company time, but whatever the reason, attendance grew. Unable to handle the load alone, we needed help. Jane

Christ, who had been one of our exercise instructors for a few years prior to Herman's, joined the LIFE ENRICHMENT Team. She, like Jen, Ralph and Janice, had shown a deeper awareness of wholistic healing than the average fitness professional. At Herman's, she grew into a phenomenal workshop instructor. Jane, like the others, benefited greatly from our strong request to become involved with Concept-Therapy. This education, with which Jane is still involved today, coupled with her unusual human insight made her an invaluable asset to both Herman's employees and us.

Feeling confident with the success of the **MBA** workshop, we were ready to introduce the mind/body connection as it related directly to health, (we had kept the health connection rather general up until then, focusing more on career, relationship and self esteem goals). We had continued with our intense study of health and felt ready to help heal Herman's. We figured if the employees liked the **MBA**, they were in for a real surprise with our wholistic health workshop. Unfortunately, the surprise was on us. We were shocked when after the first week, attendance dropped to less than half. A few weeks later attendance was down to about 20% of our original group. It was a terrible blow to our confidence and a good reason for Herman's to reconsider our quarter of a million dollar contract.

For some reason, however, no one seemed to notice our slim attendance. Why was this happening, and why wasn't anyone noticing, were two questions etched deeply into our mind. Then it dawned on us, this was our goal; perhaps not exactly as we had planned it but nonetheless just what we had asked for. We wanted to work with a dedicated group of people for a year to discover the blocks in healing and have carte blanche with which to do it. The fact that no one was monitoring what the workshops were about or how many employees attended, although quite odd, was just another aspect of our goal. Aside from the initial blow to our egos, this scenario couldn't have been more perfect.

This was not the first time and would certainly not be the last that we would have to forfeit paying homage to our egos. It is quite a task choosing between *proving* ourselves and *improving* ourselves; between looking right to the outside and living right on the inside. It is a battle that we continue to wage every day of our lives, but when we do forfeit working just for ourselves, answers come, often in a roundabout way, but they do come. What looked like a negative situation - Herman's all but rejecting our health program - was actually the path to our mission. We had dedicated ourselves to discovering why there was such a gap between our natural potential for radiant health, (ease, energy and exuberance), and our normal life of chronic problems. Thanks to the Herman's rejection, that gap was about to shorten.

Health. . . creative or curative?

Our first insight came rather quickly. In our naiveté we assumed that our enlightening health program would be flooded with eager students; after all 'health' was the number one topic on everyone's mind. Further proving how out of touch we were with society's real pulse on health, we believed that our program would be flooded with those who had some definite health problems; what better a match, sick people and a health education! Ironically, what worse of a match. Unless we were going to dispense a quick pill or verify their present condition, those who were ill had no desire to learn about health. The old paradox, 'if you want to get work done, give it to a busy person,' had a similar impact here; 'if you want to get health done - true health - give it to a healthy person.' Our health program had a very specific market, a market that up until then had been ignored, (even by us). There were too many programs and treatments for those who were *sick*, (with everything from AIDS to Z). But what about those of us who are already healthy, (relatively speaking), but want to get past - well past - the aches, pains and stresses that have become so normal? Does our potential for *wellness* stop at curing and preventing *sickness*?

Ground 0, (no serious health problem), is fine for a start, but there is a whole stretch of our health potential, 0 - 100% that has been ignored. And there is a whole segment of the population, *the not really sick but far from radiant,* that has been forgotten.

Up until then, if a person's only complaints were occasional headaches, general stiffness in their muscles and on-again-off-again fatigue, (inner stress and struggle being a given), they were considered healthy and should consider themselves lucky. We considered them neither. Although rarely publicized by our traditional health care system, (either because *they* don't know or they don't want *us* to know), freedom from even the slightest pain and flowing with outer energy and inner exuberance, is our natural state. We had found a growing number of people, sick and tired of being even a *little* sick and tired, who were ready to actualize this natural state.

This was a beginning and a good one at that. We had narrowed down the monumental health market to one specific and rather overlooked group, *the not really sick but far from radiant.* From that point on we would dedicate our programs and materials to those who were ready to experience the rarely talked about 0 - 100% realm of health; to get beyond chronic aches and pains, (no matter how slight), and experience more ease, energy and exuberance.

With an open and willing group, willing to cultivate far more than ground 0 health, the real work was about to begin. We had a rather odd task ahead of us; we had to *teach* these people while *learning* from them. We would teach *them* the general principles about health - the unlimited healing power within all of us, the mind/body connection - and then they would teach *us* what blocked these principles from working. It would prove to be a mutual healing arrangement.

We encouraged a lot of group participation in our workshops and when we listened closely to each person's questions and comments, the blocks to healing just about poured out. The first block turned out to be the most crucial and probably the most subtle. The students in the workshop agreed *as a rule* that health and illness are conditions that we ourselves create, but in the next breath they had some real *exceptions* to this rule. These exceptions included many of today's so called life threatening ills, as well as each person's own particular health problem. Most of these students believed that *other* people create their own health problems, but when it came down to the students particular problem, they had little to do with it. Genetics, environment, a screwy physiology or just bad luck were some of the defenses. We could see that this *exception to the rule* theory was not only a block for those in our workshop, but for society as a whole. In fact this belief is probably the one most responsible for society's 'sick' approach to health. To believe that human beings have creative control over their finances, relationships, self worth, success, but that health as a rule is the *exception* to this rule, is not only a block, it is pure 'B.S'!

From that point on we abbreviated society's **B**elief **S**ystems, (making an obvious point), to 'B.S.' It was the beginning of digging up what we considered the never ending 'B.S.' in society's approach to health. Our program grew into an education, both for us and our students, of the false belief systems destroying our potential for health. Presenting this education would definitely be a monumental challenge. Few people take kindly to being shown the 'B.S.' in their ideas, those in health being the most disgruntling.

'B.S.' # 1: Health is the *exception* to the rule, became the first of society's belief systems in our evolving health program. This first one, if not faced head on would keep a person in a 'sick to less sick' cycle at best, for the rest of their lives. No area of our life can change if we don't believe we have the power to change it, health being no exception to this rule. On the other hand if we *do* believe we have the power to change an area in our life, just about anything is possible. Our students agreed that this was a very simple and practical principle; they also agreed that as a society we are led to believe, (although never directly said in words), that health and health problems have little to do with a person's beliefs. Even though few people today would question the power of beliefs in affecting every area of life, in the same breath, few people would question why this power loses its power with health. We have been pounded down with the fear of illness and almost forced to surrender to the almighty 'Doc', that our own common sense is rendered a little too common to dispute the traditions of health.

We spent the next few weeks doing our version of a 'Health History;' explaining as best we could, how and why the health care system became such a 'doctatorship.' We thrashed this issue around from every conceivable angle, (described in detail in Part I of this book), exposing the untrue beliefs and unfair tactics used to keep us believing more in an artificial system than our own natural power. It was an exhausting process, (sifting through the 'B.S.' always is), but it was well worth the effort. Perhaps for the first time in their lives, these students had more faith in their own healing power than fear of health problems. Although all of us would have to put this faith to the test every time we got ill or started to fear illness, what had just been gained or regained could never be lost. We all had regained a trust in our own inner power to create our inner and outer life, and health would never again be the 'exception' to this rule.

The *exception to the rule* belief was the first, perhaps most damaging 'B.S.' but it was only the beginning. In our excitement over proving that a person *can* have creative control over their health, we neglected one fundamental point; did they *want* to? For the masses, being in creative control of one's own health was considered a major headache. No wonder Herman's medical claims had risen while attendance in our health workshop had fallen. Why take responsibility for health, (beyond eating and exercising well), when society has set up a system to do it for us? The thousand and one health insurance companies all promise, (for a fee of course), to 'insure' our health. The drug companies continue to force the 'pill theory' down our throats. We are lead to believe that an outside system can take 'care' of our health. But if this were true, considering today's billion dollar Health Care System, shouldn't we have at least million dollar health?

We as a society have been well marketed into believing that health is a *product we can buy*. The truth is that health is a *by product* of our thoughts, beliefs and lifestyle. Believing that we can buy health is just more 'B.S.' Unfortunately it is the widely accepted 'B.S.' Taking actual responsibility for our health, beginning with healing the 'B.S.' within, is shunned like the plague. This is especially true when we are promised a future cure for most of the worlds ills. But we have to face the fact that our billion dollar drug industry is sold to us through million dollar ad campaigns. Dare we ask the question, "Are we being sold on the wonders of modern *medicine* through the wonders of modern *marketing*?"

Although our society pushes the 'healthy lifestyle' mentality, in reality it is the 'wait and sick' one that prevails. Few will deny that they wait until they get sick before knocking down the doors for health, the doors of the nearest doctor. While a doctor may be able to *relieve* certain symptoms, until the sick beliefs are healed, (*our* responsibility), the same problem or something worse, returns again and again. To believe that anyone else can do it for us, is just more 'B.S.' or **'B.S.' # 2: Our Health Care System *can* and *should* take responsibility for our health.**

Our Health Care System *can't* and *shouldn't* take responsibility for our health. This is the truth and later in this book it will be explained why this is also to our greatest advantage. However, without an understanding, this news could be a major blow. Finding out that our sacred Health Care System - our other 'God' - is *not* God, is no easy pill to swallow. Taking true responsibility for one's life never is, health being no exception to this rule.

Our workshop at Herman's pivoted between truth and 'B.S.' Although our students never knew it, we presented the truth about health while waiting for the 'B.S.' to be revealed; ironically this always happened when we least expected it.

'B.S.' # 3: popped up during one of the exercises in our workshop. We asked the students to write down their health goal; a standard procedure for attaining any goal. Expecting to hear the students describe their health *dreams,* we were shocked to hear more about their health *nightmares.* This exercise said it all about society's rather sick picture of health. All of us are so hammered each day with the fear of illness - the media doing most of the pounding - that we talk about health in terms of *not getting sick.* This standard is as limiting as equating success with not being a failure, or worse yet, equating a good relationship with not being abused. No one in their right mind would equate these opposites, yet for reasons explained throughout the workshop and throughout this book, health has become the exception to this rule.

Not realizing the rather sick slant to their goals, the students related health with more *desperation* than *inspiration.* Avoiding one of the 'top ten illnesses' was far more common than creating a state of ease, energy and exuberance. Some did write the standard health clichés; *sound mind and body, feeling good, lots of energy,* were some of the bright spots. But when asked to really describe these clichés, how it would *feel* to feel this way, the students were stumped. It became obvious that most people have a clearer picture of what they *don't* want, (or what they fear), than what they *do* want. It doesn't take a genius to see that focusing on and fearing what we don't want, (warning signs included), is just asking for trouble.

Unfortunately, our natural instinct to envision vibrant, energetic and joyful health has all but withered away. It has been squelched by a health care system that equates *not being too sick* - headaches, allergies and other not so serious problems accepted - with good health. Human potential is encouraged to climbing to the top of

Mt. Everest, but as far as climbing to our potential for *health*, we are kept flat on the ground.

While our students did come up with a grander, richer vision for health, (taking more time and effort than any of us had expected), we came up with **'B.S.' # 3: Good health means not being sick.** Just like the previous two, this 'B.S.' could not be further from the truth. We are all entitled to a richness of health, far beyond avoiding *poor* health. Good health starts with ease, energy and an exuberance for life, and works up from there. First we must heal our health *vision* if we can ever expect to heal our health *condition.*

No one was more amazed at the way the workshop was evolving than we were. What began as an introduction to the mind/body connection and the unlimited healing power within, turned into an expose of the *blocks* to these principles. Then again, this was what we originally wanted to happen.

Assuming that we were finished with the 'B.S.' (the last three had more than rattled our brains) we moved on to another principle. Up until then we had related the idea of health to the *body;* God knows their was more than enough 'B.S.' just with *physical* health. And Herman's employees were in need of true physical health at the very least, but there was more. Since Herman's had become the microcosm of society as a whole, what was true for the former was equally true for the latter. Ever since we began with Herman's, we observed a particular kind of suffering and need for healing that went deeper than the body. Mental and spiritual wholeness, the real meaning of health, were far from the normal state. Whenever we had an intimate conversation with someone, they poured their hearts out, hearts that were filled with pain and frustration. Again we took this to symbolize society as a whole. And once again we realized another hole in one of our traditional systems. This time the hole was the lack of *wholeness* in our approach to health.

Physical health is so important, especially to someone who is ill. But to assume that it is the 'be all and end all' of life, the area in which we should devote billions of dollars and most of our attention is just more 'B.S.' Health, true health is about healing the *whole* person; hence the meaning of *holistic* health, (we spell it *wholistic* to be more distinct). A person is truly healthy when they are *physically* full of ease and energy, *mentally* flowing with peace and *spiritually* exuberant and grounded. This may sound like a lot to hope for, but like radiant physical health, radiant mental and spiritual health are the natural states. They are natural, however, only when we follow the laws of our nature, not necessarily the beliefs of our society.

All the great minds of society, beginning with Hippocrates, (the Father of 'Medicine'), taught about healing the whole *being,* not the whole *body* as has become the accepted practice. We have come to believe that putting 100% of our focus on 30% of our nature, the body, is an intelligent approach. But it doesn't take a rocket scientist to realize that these odds can never be in our favor. From mania with drugs and physical treatments to obsession with nutrition, our health care system tries to artificially create what is already natural to our being. The whole point of health is and always had been, (until we became so 'high tech'), to heal and fulfill the *whole being.* Our students wholeheartedly agreed with this wholistic principle. It took several weeks in the workshop, (and several chapters in this book), to discover *how* to heal and fulfill the physical, mental and spiritual aspects of our being. Talk about dedication, these students worked painstakingly at this new education while watching hundreds of their coworkers line up for their annual cholesterol screening; an event that many believed satisfied their health requirements for the year.

It was frustrating to watch Herman's, (and society as a whole), become fascinated with their cholesterol reading while barely noticing this 'whole' other approach to health, but it did yield **'B.S.' # 4: Healing is *from* the body and *for* the body.** Was there no end to the 'B.S.'? Health is neither *of* the body, (the mind/body connection proves that point), nor just *for* the body. As long as society continues to focus on what is good for the body while ignoring what is needed for the mind and the inner self or soul, living happily and healthily ever after will never pass the fairy tale stage.

What began as a nine week workshop turned into one that was now in its ninth month. We had no idea that there would be so much 'B.S.' about health or that it would take so long to get past it. The belief systems we had shared over the many months, (society's 'B.S.'), were universal in nature. Now, nine months later we were finally ready to get a bit more *personal.* We knew from personal experience that everyone had their own personal brand of beliefs that were either supporting or sabotaging their life, health no longer being the exception to this rule. Although we were a little more knowledgeable about these beliefs than the universal ones that took nine months to discover, we still lacked some valuable insights. These insights came during what we called our 'One on One Goal Consulting.' Many employees preferred these private sessions over a group workshop; they were not comfortable revealing their deep feelings to a whole group. For some reason they sure felt comfortable revealing them to us.

Other than posing questions, we mostly listened while people talked and *talked,* anywhere from 20 minutes to as much as an hour. The goals ranged from wanting a better self to wanting better health, those on health being the most crucial to us. Once again it was a mutual healing arrangement; we helped the employees realize their own healing power and they helped us realize the 'B.S.' now on a personal level, that blocked this power. Issues like need for attention, feeling unworthy of great health, harboring deep guilt and feeling the need to be punished, (sickness and pain being a standard punishment), and on and on *ad nauseam;* it was really sick what unknowingly we do to our health. And as usual there was far more 'B.S.' than we had ever imagined. Part II of this book gives a thorough explanation.

Our greatest 'health breakthrough,' the belief that probably binds us tightest to our chronic problems, was so subtle it almost passed us right by. For so long we had heard people, (ourselves many times as well), precede an ill with the word, "my." From "my backaches," to "my bursitis," there was rarely a chronic condition that didn't have a binding "my" before it. The major cause of the chronic problems with our body was right under our own nose. Unfortunately it was either too subtle or too common - who doesn't have a *my condition?* - to make the connection. Fortunately for our students and our clients we did. For many, (us included), this one insight led to the decrease or in some cases total disappearance of a life long battle with chronic pain. Even though a tremendous breakthrough, without the nine months of work, this bond idea with the body would have gone in one ear and out the other. It took all that time to regain the faith in healing, faith that had previously been lost in all the 'B.S.'.

Although this ever evolving health program had now gone on for almost a year, we were not quite ready to call it a day. There was one more principle that was so crucial to our well being and at the same time so confused with misinformation. We had begun the healing cycle with the body. We were going to end it with the self.

True Self Healing had long since become the focus and the purpose of our work and our lives. We knew that this principle needed much clearing up. Many people believe the idea of 'self healing' means that we have to heal our self, all by our self. True Self Healing does not mean healing *by* our self, but rather healing *of* our self. Healing the pains and ills of the body is a wonderful freedom. But until we heal the pains and ills of the self, allowing the Real Divine Self to flow through, we are not free at all; not physically for long, and not mentally or spiritually for sure. We felt obligated to encourage a person to dedicate their lives to this idea of Real Self healing. It was a process that there was not time to cultivate during the workshop, (management wanted their conference room back already!) We suggested a Concept-Therapy class to really explain this Real Self principle. God knows these people were more than prepared to grasp the advanced internal education offered through Concept-Therapy.

The end of this whole-istic health workshop really meant the beginning for all of us. As our health program ended, there was yet another monumental task ahead of us. We had to find a way to scale down a health program that took almost a year to present into a book that wouldn't take a year to read! Three years later, the task was completed. **"Health Beyond *Belief*,"** a book definitely true to its title, begins to heal the sick beliefs standing between us and our birthright for true health.

Twelve years in the making, this book more than satisfies the purpose and the objectives that we had set over a dozen years ago. We have witnessed the principles in **"Health Beyond *Belief*"** awaken greater physical, mental and spiritual health than we and our students ever dreamed possible. And considering the almost impossible standards to which we are bound, (twelve years of research before we felt right to write), this was a dream that almost didn't come true!

PART I

Beyond Society's Belief Systems - 'B.S.' about Health

Talk about an idea whose time has come! We are finally turning our backward approach to life, most specifically health, inside out. Our inner beliefs, once laughed at as an intelligent solution to problems, are now honored as the cause and cure of every area of our life; health being no exception.

The 20th century will mark the greatest rise in <u>outward</u> progress, physically and technologically in history. Isn't it ironic that the last decade of this century will mark the crucial shift toward <u>inward</u> progress, mentally and spiritually as well?

Releasing our unlimited power within especially for health, is as natural to human beings as breathing. The only thing that separates us from our natural state of radiant health is the preprogrammed <u>B</u>elief <u>S</u>ystems - 'B.S.' - fed into our minds and into our spirits. Getting beyond this 'B.S.', beginning with Society's unique brand, is an idea whose time has definitely come!

"Hark, I hear a Cannon!"

"Hark, I hear a cannon! Hark, I hear a cannon!" the proud actor repeated. Given one line in a play, he was going to get it perfect.
Obsessed with sounding great, this actor never gave much thought
to what the line really meant. The day of the performance, the
sound of a cannon blasted through the theater cueing him to say his
line. Startled by the sound, instead of saying his line, the well intended actor turned to the director and said, "What the hell was
that!"

We have repeated that story in workshops for over a decade. So
subtle a point, it takes a person awhile to get it, but once realized,
the analogy to life is powerful. We as a society have become so familiar with repeating information we have heard or read, that too
often we accept it on blind faith. We forget to question the logic of
it; does it make sense? We see a new health warning on TV, read
about a breakthrough in the newspaper, hear a health debate on a
talk show, listen to a theory from our neighbors, remember an old
wives tale from our grandmothers or get a diagnosis from our
plumber who had the same condition, and bam! these ideas become
our facts. If these so called 'facts' had to do with gardening, beauty
care or buying a car, they would not really impact the quality of our
life. But since the majority of these 'facts' have to do with health,
they not only impact but often *define* the quality of our life. Scan-
ning these so called facts, the bad news is that they paint a gloomy,
often hopeless picture of health. The good news is that most, if not
all of these so called facts are 'B.S.'

Belief Systems - 'B.S.'

With the exception of our divine nature, Belief Systems - 'B.S.' - are
the most powerful aspect of our being. It is so mind boggling that
this most powerful part of our being (also referred to as the
mind/body connection), is all but ignored when it comes to 'real
life'. Where in all of our 12 - 20 years of schooling did we have a

course on inner beliefs? When was the last time a health professional trying to discover the cause of our health problem question
our beliefs about it? The ignorance of our inner beliefs solves the
mystery as to why the same problems - chronic headaches, constant
stress, relationship conflicts, career mishaps, self doubt - plague our
life year after year.

On first glance, one would find it hard to believe that our society
has ignored inner beliefs. Isn't the *mind/body connection* on everyone's minds these days? Hasn't *mental imagery* become a practical
path to success? Doesn't the medical society accept *stress* as the
basis of most ills? Aren't *self help* books becoming almost as popular as the romance novels? With all the hullabaloo about the mind,
you'd think we would have this mind/body thing knocked. Well,
think again. While there has never before been so much talk about
how we can use our mind to heal our life, the effects don't seem to
match the effort. Many of us do accept the mind/body connection,
mental imagery, stress management and self help, but in the end
genuine, lasting life improvements are minimal if at all. Does this
mean that this mind/body thing is really a bunch of 'B.S.'? Yes, but
not the kind of 'B.S.' we think.

Belief Systems - 'B.S.' go far deeper than casual mind/body conversations or occasional dabs with mental imagery. They are as
powerful as they are subtle. Belief Systems - 'B.S.' are preprogrammed ideas, (acquired and inherited basically from childhood),
upon which our life is based. For example, if we have bought the
belief that money is hard to come by, until this belief is changed,
money will be hard to come by. If we have the belief that we are a
whiz at math, as long as we have that belief, we will be. So far, this
principle of beliefs sounds logical and true; few people today would
dispute its authenticity, at least in theory.

No matter how much we read and discuss the power of mind over
matter, again and again the "Hark, I hear a cannon!" syndrome
takes over when it comes to real life. All too often, we look at

something negative that is happening to us and think, "what the heck is that?" We genuinely feel that we weren't thinking about struggling with money, gaining weight, fighting with our mate or having a headache; in fact these thoughts never even crossed our minds. In one sense we are right, these thoughts never did cross our minds. That is the beauty (or the danger) of beliefs. They are so conditioned, so subtle and so automatic that they can completely run our life without the least thought on our part. We can be sure that any condition in our life or any feeling in our hearts that occurs over and over, *apparently* with no forethought on our part is rooted in a belief.

This book will help us in revealing and healing the insidious beliefs that run and often ruin our life; those about health being the most crucial. Belief Systems are discussed so much in this book, they are abbreviated as 'B.S.' More to the point however, we refer to Belief Systems as 'B.S.' because no matter how real they may seem, or how long we have been run by them, at bottom, all Belief Systems are 'B.S.'

While it may seem personally insulting that the majority of our life is built on 'B.S.', this is the good news. Beliefs can be changed, facts can't. So how do we know whether conditions in our life, conditions that we desperately want to change, are built on facts or 'B.S.'? The distinction is fairly simple; if something is a fact for *us,* it must be a fact for *all.* That tremendously narrows down the scope of facts, particularly those that we have thought could never change. We must eat to live - fact. As we get older, our metabolism slows down and more of what we eat turns to fat - 'B.S.' If only one person stays in the same lean shape at eighty as they did at thirty, it is true and just as possible for all of us. If only one person healed themselves of a chronic ill (and there is at least one person who has healed themselves of every ill there is), it is true and just as possible for all of us. And if only one person lived a long, radiantly healthy life, we all can. There will be one major point stressed over

and over in this book; the only thing that stands between us and a
fully functional life is the 'B.S.'

Getting in touch with our inner beliefs so that we can heal our outer
life is a lifetime process. Anytime we feel stuck in a negative feeling or bound to a negative condition, it is the belief that first must
be changed; that is what is meant by creative control. In fact,
changing the beliefs in our mind is often the last control that we
take, yet the only control we really have.

Beliefs are subtle but powerful; they tie us up in knots until we are
so caught in our own 'B.S.' that we *believe* it is who we are. Beliefs do not come with a protective warning that says, "These are
preprogrammed ideas and not absolute facts; do not allow them to
limit and bind you." Because we have never been taught about the
power of beliefs, instead of thinking, "I have a *belief* that I am
sick," we go right for the jugular and emphatically proclaim, "I *am*
sick." Regardless of the circumstance, once it becomes an *I am, it
is.*

There is an upside to these beliefs. They have a total equal opportunity policy. Beliefs cannot discriminate between negative and
positive, one is no more difficult for a belief than the other. The
prevailing belief unfortunately is that the good things in life are far
more difficult, if not impossible, than the problems. The truth is
that wonderful relationships are just as easy for a belief to attract as
painful relationships. Abundance takes no more effort for a belief
than struggle and hardship. And depending on our belief, we can
just as naturally radiate with health as we can suffer with illness.
Again, just more 'B.S.' to be healed. That belief may seem like
'B.S.' right now, but take heart; as this book unfolds, what seemed
like 'B.S.' will prove to be truth and more crucially, what seemed
like truth will prove to be 'B.S.'

Until we sharpen our inner vision, we are virtually blind to our own
'B.S.' Belief Systems are so instinctive that until this happens, we

rarely see them coming. But if directed correctly this can be to our great advantage. Beliefs are on automatic pilot for the purpose of convenience. Who wants to think about how to drive (like when we first learned), every time we get in the car. Talk about an automatic belief! We can now listen to a tape, drink a cup of coffee and calm a crying child all without missing our exit. Is this juggling act really so easy? No, it is just a preprogrammed habit, a part of who we are. The same is true with chronic problems in our life. Over and over, seemingly without warning, we automatically find ourselves with the same mess. Whether it is the same allergy or the same argument with our spouse, when we are honest and in touch, it is not difficult to dig up a belief behind it all. All of the great minds have proved that we can move mountains by changing our thinking. By the same token because of a stubborn belief, the tiniest of molehills can keep us imprisoned for years. From chronic headaches to financial struggles, even hanging on to the same extra five pounds for years falls into this category; our outer life is just mirroring our inner beliefs. The freedom begins when we realize that we have no chronic problems, only chronic 'B.S.'!

Haven't you always wondered why two people with exactly the same actions come up with totally different results? Take two people with exactly the same physiology and you will find that one has chronic indigestion no matter what they eat while the other can eat like a horse and feel great. Why haven't more people asked why? Sales managers have been stymied by some salespeople who can soar to the top in a short time while others, with the same amount of appointments never make their quota. To this day, Doreen's mother creates a heavenly quiche while Doreen can follow the exact same recipe only to create a flat frisbee. While frantically searching for the missing ingredient, the realization came that it is the belief or vision of the cook that makes the difference between a masterpiece and a mess. Doreen's mothers always expects a masterpiece while Doreen knows that she is playing with fire every time she cooks a quiche. Both beliefs are right.

Somewhere along the line, Pat accepted the fact (really the belief) that if something were mechanical, she couldn't do it. In fact, (another characteristic of beliefs) Pat's extremely intelligent mind goes almost blank when someone tries to explain how to operate a machine. When she had to record tapes for exercise class, she felt like she had all thumbs and no brains. Later on, the VCR was like an alien from space, (she never could set the clock right), and it took her a month to get the big idea of the fax. She still can't understand why someone on the other end can receive a fax when *her machine* is out of paper! Interestingly though, Pat can beat the pants off of anyone in Trivial Pursuit but needs her six year old daughter to explain to her how to work the VCR! It makes no sense but that is the whole point; beliefs have no sense, they just do exactly what they are or were told.

When it was established that this book had to be written on computer so that it wouldn't take three *more* years to complete, the shaking and sweating began; but there would be no way out of this one. Sick and tired of all the anxiety and fear over anything that had more than an on / off switch, and wanting desperately to get this book out, (more than even the risk of failure), to write this book Pat broke right through her own 'B.S.' The belief about the 'mechanical monster' still comes up, but now that she has faced it and continues to work at changing it, the computer was mastered and this book was completed.

It doesn't take a genius to realize there is more to outer results than meets the eye. We can't see them but our beliefs predetermine our future outcomes. This is not easy to accept, especially when it comes to looking at our problems, but this is good news. Logic dictates that if the *problem* is within our own head, then so is the *power*. Too many people live under the universal principle of, "hey, this problem isn't *my* fault." But when we absolve ourselves from responsibility, in the same breath we forfeit any power to change. If we deny one, we reject both. Denying our own beliefs at the expense of retaining creative power is one of the main reasons that we

do not get from life what we want. The price of pride over principle is far to high.

While beliefs create *every* area of our life, the rest of this book will
be talking about the 'B.S.' that comes between us and our birthright
for radiant health. And that 'B.S.' runs deep. Think about that
statement. Unfortunately, when it comes to health, society has
conditioned us *not* to think. We have been subtly taught that outside experts like doctors, the media, drug companies, even the tab-
loids know what is best or worst for our health. That is pure 'B.S.'
Yes, we can partner with a doctor or anyone that can elevate our
health, health is a partnership not a *doctator*ship. Nobody is more
of an expert when it comes to our own health than we are. And
that is no 'B.S.'!

The purpose of this book is to get us to rethink in our *minds* about
totally putting the health of our *bodies* in someone else's *hands*.
Health beyond *Belief* is about regaining creative control over our
health. And when we do, health as we have never experienced it
before will be ours. Part I of this book exposes and heals the false
Belief Systems, in other words, the 'B.S.' that society has fed us
about health:

(1) Health is the exception to the rule.
(2) Our health care system *can* and *should*
be responsible for our health.
(3) Good health means 'not being sick'.
(4) Healing is *from* the body and *for* the body.

But take heed. . . Belief Systems are as subtle as they are treacherous; they write out the script to our life and before even batting an
eye, we are playing the part to the hilt. To insist that we are above
the 'B.S.', that we know our own mind and are in full control of it,
is not only dangerous, it is 'B.S.' Pride aside, let's take this opportunity offered to meticulously see where, not *if*, we are bound by
limiting, false belief systems. Read closely, absorb gradually. Let

the ideas roll around in the mind for awhile before agreeing or disagreeing. The main goal of our own 'B.S.' is to fight to be right.
But this is not an I.Q. test. We are dealing with health; it is not
about being *right*, it is about being *well*.

'B.S.' # 1:
Health is the 'exception' to the rule.

We have been subtly taught to live by two sets of rules; one for health and one for all other areas of life. We have been conditioned to accept that we have creative control over our life, our careers, relationships, our self esteem but for some strange reason, health has become the 'exception' to that rule.

This fundamental 'B.S.' that health obeys a set of rules and laws to which we human beings are not privy, is more responsible for the lack of radiant health than all the germs on earth. Once a person accepts the belief that health is something that happens *to* them, instead of being created *through* them, fear runs the heart and hopelessness the head. A person with the mind set that health or health problems just mysteriously appear, surrenders their God given right to grow in radiant health. It is much more tragic for a person to have a sick belief than a sick body. A sick body can be healed, but if the mind is sick with dis-ease beliefs, the body will heal from one dis-ease or one episode of a dis-ease only to inevitably relapse at a later date or come down with another dis-ease. Without healing the sick beliefs in the mind, we remain in this sad sick cycle.

Keep in mind we are talking about creating a state of radiant or fully functional health. Today's traditional health care system, along with all its 'B.S.' may be valuable for those people with major health problems. The traditional system cannot and does not venture into the realm of *radiant* health. And it is society's 'B.S.', particularly that health has its own set of rules that's been keeping us from this radiance. *Until now.*

Society's subtle teaching that health is the *exception* to the rules of life is only 'B.S.' # 1. Make no mistake, this belief ultimately decides whether we have creative control over our health or become a victim to every whim of nature, God and government. This is far from the first book to explain the unlimited healing power within, a frequently quoted author, Ralph Waldo Trine wrote about this power back in 1908. In his book "In Tune with the Infinite" he wrote, "In the degree that you realize the Infinite Spirit of Life is within, and actualize your latent powers, you will exchange disease for ease and suffering and pain for abounding health." No, this is not the first book to tell why the truths of the ages have lost out to the 'B.S.' of the times. Until it finally hits us that we have been bamboozled into believing that health and health problems obey a set of rules all their own, that they come and go more by their own accord than our control, (we would never buy that 'B.S.' with any other area of our life), there isn't a chance in health that things will ever improve. And there is no exception to that rule. On the other hand, the hand that we finally have a chance to play, as we face the fact that only 'B.S.' can keep us from abounding health, there is no limit to the possibilities.

So how did health become the exception to the rule? By ignoring three major principles of life:

1. Positive Thinking
2. Personal and Spiritual Power
3. The right to Question, Think and Disagree

1. Positive Thinking

We as a society have been trained to believe that our Health Care System takes a most *positive* approach to health. Its ceaseless efforts, (never does a day go by without a major health breakthrough in the news) its caring words, "we are devoted to you and your family's health" seem to be as positive as it gets. But motives can be misleading and caring can be deceiving. To assume that our Health Care System focuses mostly on the positive aspects of our health could not be further from the truth.

It may be unsettling to discover that the system which ranks right up there with 'mother', (our Health Care System), might be *contributing* to our ills rather than curing them. This kind of statement can rock us to the core, but keep this idea in mind, we are not suggesting to eliminate this traditional system, just *illuminate* it; fill it with the light of truth. We are not saying to drop all our past ideas about health and blindly accept all these new ones. Rather, listen to the logic of these new ideas and if they make sense, and *only* if they make sense, try them out. Unlike the new drug treatments that we are asked to try everyday, these ideas are natural, have no sick side effects and open us to the power that runs the entire universe.

Now, let's talk logic. If there has ever been a revolution of *positive* thinking, it is today. Teachers, preachers and parents, when dealing with a goal or a problem, reinforce the power of positive thoughts. Coaches from Peewee football to Olympic training, know that *positive* visualization, (seeing the desired outcome), makes the difference between a good athlete and a superstar. Motivating speakers talking about financial prosperity, relationship harmony, self esteem and weight loss lecture that above all else, a *positive* self image over education or determination sets the stage for success.

A negative approach to positive thinking

No intelligent person today would argue that focusing on the positive desired outcome is the pivot point between success and failure. We all know that. Why then have we made the fatal mistake of viewing health as the *exception* to this rule? It is subtle and often missed completely, but when we take away all the smiling faces in commercials and heart warming pictures on billboards, the real message in today's Health Care System is far less than positive. It suggests a grim, painful, often fatalistic view of health. Not in so many words, of course, but definitely in so many ways. Newspaper headlines, often front page news explode with the new virus coming our way. Statistics on the escalating odds of us 'catching' one of the top ten illnesses scare us to death. We are told to have hope (although its track record leaves much to be desired), that one day a cure will come. Is that part of the same fairy tale that suggests one day our prince will come?

Everyday, whether we are listening to our neighbor or reading another All-star benefit for the latest sick charity, society forces us to obsess over health, even though we possess an unlimited healing power. There is not a whole lot of press on our healing power, however, is there? The statement is clear; focus on what could go wrong with the body, fear the likelihood of getting ill, and reinforce our *powerlessness* over this whole health situation. Some positive message!

It is sad to admit but society does take a negative approach to positive thinking as far as health is concerned. Anytime we focus on the *problem* - or whatever it is - and ignore our inner creative *power*, we have taken a negative approach to the principle of positive thinking. Regardless of how much our 'health' (sickness) experts may try to convince us otherwise, health is no exception to this rule.

Before exposing more on the 'B.S.' that Health is the *exception* to the rule, understand that this negative realization is a positive step. We are realizing that today's 'problems' with health is in our *approach*, not our *ability*.

We have the power, it is our focus of this power that needs to be healed. We have been victims of this negative approach to positive health. It would be almost impossible to live in this society amid the monumental propaganda ('B.S.') about health injected into our heads through the most hypnotic suggestions and be immune to it.

As we face the 'B.S.' however, and reinforce the unlimited power within us (the goal of this book), we open up to physical, mental and spiritual **Health beyond** *Belief.* Be aware; even with the promise of radiant health, when it comes to questioning the American Health Care System, a system that ranks right up there with Mother, Apple Pie and the Olympics, the skepticism and devotion run deep.

So, how did we get so devoted to a system that discourages the principle of life from entering the practice of health? It wasn't easy.

Bound through anger and fear

Before they have heard the full story, many people take personal offense at the suggestion that our sacred Health Care System might be misleading us. When we suggest that there might be a better way, you would think we were denouncing a person's religion! Unfortunately, in our faithful homage we may be unknowingly viewing doctors, drugs and the Health Care System as another God. Out of fear (it is a sacrilege to question the mysteries of the medical profession, you know!), many of us accept as gospel the words of our doctor, TV 'health' expert or magazine article. Desperately we hope that if we do what we are told we will be sent to 'health heaven.' As is often the case with religion, we are bound to our traditional Health Care System by anger and fear; anger that any scrutiny of this system is viewed as a personal attack and fear that if we question or refute the accepted practices, "God is gonna get us," with disease as our punishment. We have been well trained.

The tide of holistic healing, although very much in the public eye, has yet to turn. In our early days, we quickly learned that sharing these truths with others was the fastest way to start an argument. We used to get on our soap box and 'educate' our friends and family on the negative aspects of their beloved health system. Needless to say, we lost friends and strained family relationships. We learned two things though; never offer health advice unless asked and when asked, realize that anger and fear are running the show. Learning where and when to talk about this emotional subject is one thing, but we never compromise these health principles in our hearts or our homes. We and our principles have certainly been put to the test. New reports on the latest disease and the likelihood of '1 out of 9 of us getting it,' are broadcast everyday. People all around us talk about their newest virus. The American Medical Association, (our *other* house of worship) often declares that holistic health, the mind/body connection and the unlimited healing power within are all 'B.S.', so how do we avoid being sucked in by such well positioned fear? Through the only two resources that can overpower our fear in health; logic and experience. As we reinforce the logic of health as a creative process (no different than any other area of life) and experience this process working over and over again, the fear is gone.

The logic of it all

Logic, the science of reliable reasoning, is one of our greatest tools. As human beings, we are gifted with the ability to reason on life situations, to see the simple logic of it all. In fact, it really all comes down to very *simple logic*; as you sow, you reap. Literally or symbolically, we plant a seed in the ground (whether it is the ground of the earth or the ground of the mind) and there is no mystery as to what will grow. As long as the ground, (matter or mind), is *fertile*, *frequently weeded* and *nurtured* - our only responsibilities - the perfect crop is assured. No one in their right mind would question this *logical process* in farming, or with any 'crop' desired in life. Why then, have we allowed *health* to be the exception to this logical rule? Does the rule really say, 'As you sow, you reap; except in health?' Of course not. Then how can it be logical to sow fears about illness, thoughts about the new virus in town or conversations about all our aches and pains and still expect health? It can't.

With logic and without fear, we can ask ourselves some powerful questions. Why with health and illness does the process of logic lose out to luck, punishment or some mysterious force beyond our control? Does it really make logical sense that the Supreme Being that created us would grant us full creative license in all areas of life *except* health? What could be the meaning of "being God's privileged children," and in the same breath be damned to a life of fighting and fearing illness? It is time we put some intelligent reasoning to these illogical and damaging beliefs. Logic says that if human beings are given creative control over their lives, then believing that health is the exception to this rule no longer makes reasonable sense, in other words, it is just more 'B.S.' In our own lives, logic is what allowed us to slowly eliminate the fear and mystery surrounding our own health problems. This logical reasoning that health obeys the same rules as any other goal in life proved to us that connecting with our own unlimited healing power is *possible*. Actual experience with this power convinced us that it was not only possible but *do-able*.

From logic to living

Seeing the logic in healing, (when was the last time we heard the words 'logic' and 'healing' in the same sentence?) begins stripping away the God awful fear of illness dyed into our brains. Fear of illness just naturally fades away as the confidence in the simple logic of health grows. Logic gets us going in the right direction. But *living* it keeps us there, forever.

We have personally experienced the magic of our own healing power so many times and through so many 'ills'. Conditions that might seem insignificant if not impossible to others - healing a cold in a matter of minutes, eliminating years of migraines in what seemed like overnight, and most importantly, watching the miracle of this healing power in our own children - are proof positive that society's negative approach to health has got to change.

Everyone has experiences of being part of the creative process in healing, we are doing it all the time although we are not aware of it. Some of us have just decided to consciously watch it work. In our own lives, we have lost count of how many times we have watched in awe the healing power at work, though some instances are still quite vivid.

One night about 2:00 a.m. Doreen woke up with all the signs of a cold and sore throat. As always, she made a cup of hot tea, the best remedy for her years of colds and sore throats. Doreen knew that the tea (with honey and lemon, of course), would soothe her symptoms. She sat at the kitchen table, tea in hand, and decided for the first time not to give in to the pain and fear. She relaxed her mind and body totally and just let her body do whatever it needed, pain and all.

Too tired to fight it, she just allowed the power within to do its natural healing job. Feeling much better she went back to bed. The next day she was free of all pain and symptom with more energy than she had in awhile. A little skeptical, she thought it must have been the hot tea that did the trick. Walking into the kitchen she noticed that the tea that had 'healed' her, had never been touched.

What was it that healed Doreen? Was it some mysterious coincidence or was it mind over matter? In her mind, it really didn't matter. She knew that she could tap into a healing power that defied time and condition. From then on, Doreen would find a way to experience these 'mini-miracles' on a regular basis.

Our profession allows us the opportunity to see this healing power work with others. Many times we have seen symptoms and problems disappear just from a good talk. After being given permission to express their feelings or renew their faith in themselves, so many people have stood in awe as their tension, fear and pain melt away.

Is this power fool proof? Yes. Are we? Not always. We still have unhealed beliefs that cause us to direct this power against ourselves. But the more we can see the logic of this power and the more experience we gain from using it in our lives, the more faith we build. Who needs the fear of illness ringing in our heads or chronic pain and discomfort, (even if it isn't fatal, it certainly kills our day), when we are privy to a power that just waits for the chance to heal. This new insight does not mean we should abandon all traditional health practices; they have their *place*. But contrary to popular belief, they cannot *take the place* of connecting with the source of all healing, the power within. By now it should be no secret that this first 'B.S.', health is the exception to the rules of logic, has a tough grip on us.

This section began with exposing how our society accepts the principle of positive thinking as the foundation of life and yet takes a negative approach when it comes to health. The first negative was that our traditional health system keeps us *bound through anger and fear*. Even when traditional treatments have only marginal benefits and the side effects are often as bad as the problem, many still find it difficult to try 'alternative' methods. Subliminally we are kept bound through a 'do or die' suggestion that implies if we do take a more wholistic approach, we could be risking our life or the life of our family. Now who wants that kind of guilt on their conscience? With the fear of death planted in our minds, many of us remain loyal to a system that doesn't work. Fear can keep us obedient but it cannot keep us well. No matter how justified, fear on a regular basis has harmful effects. Ask a psychologist. Any system to which we are bound by fear depresses our entire being and a depressed being cannot be well.

It is quite a realization to see that our Health Care System uses a powerful marketing tool, the 'fear of death,' to keep us customers for life. It takes an inwardly strong person to reevaluate such a traditional system and to question how much this system really has our best interests in mind. When we do shake off the victim role that we have been unknowingly playing, however, and take up our rightful place and responsibility as creators of health, (the fear of our Health Care System and the purpose of this book), that inward strength becomes available to us.

If we can stay open to the logic and truth of healing, see the 'B.S.' in today's practices for what it really is, *in time,* our life and our health will rise to radiant levels. Along the way, however, we may have to contend with the condemnation of today's health fundamentalists, those family, friends and health professionals who will take personal offense at *our* nontraditional approach to health.

Unfortunately many people feel risking the wrath of others is too high a price to pay, even for their own health. Fortunately, there are more and more exceptions to this rule today. Now that the 'new' holistic health education is available, (although it has been around 2,000 years or more), it is not so anti- American to question the traditional system. And now that a well hidden principle called *logic* has entered on the scene, the 'power of life' within us will begin to melt the 'fear of death' that used to bind us. There is more to this negative approach to positive thinking when it comes to health. This next illogical approach may just be the crux of the whole health problem in our society.

A sick focus

We began this section with the fact that focusing on the *positive* - positive thinking, positive visualizing, a positive self image - is the ultimate factor between success and failure. This principle has always been accepted and practiced by the greatest minds, past and present, so we shall not reprove the point. However, there is a point that cannot be stressed enough. Focusing our God given power on what we *want* as opposed to focusing it on what we *don't* want, or what could go wrong, doesn't change loyalties when it comes to health. In other words, if we want to become an Olympic skier, memorizing the seven warning signs of potential failure, checking every few minutes to see if a warning sign has appeared, or listening to statistics on how many ski disasters occur every day, would be ludicrous and highly counterproductive. Why then is memorizing the seven warning signs of every illness imaginable, checking our body regularly to see if a warning has appeared yet or listening to statistics on how many health disasters will occur this year, seen as a 'positive approach' to health? Only with health can we get away with taking such a negative approach and expect a positive result! Do we really believe that hearing the grave fore-cast of ills every time we open a newspaper, turn on the TV news or read a health article in a magazine, is a healthy approach? Simple logic tells us that filling our minds with vivid pictures of the symptoms of pain and sickness is just asking for trouble. Even a beginner to the mind/body connection would expect such a sick focus to push these images right through to our bodies. Have we completely ignored the irrefutable *power of suggestion* just because we are talking about health? How quickly does the flu or a virus spread through a city like wildfire within days of its broadcast on TV or as front page news? It is no coincidence that sales of sinus tablets and cold relief medications skyrocket the day that the cold and allergy season announcement is made. Imagine how many other illnesses, chronic and serious have been spread through the power of suggestion. Does this mean to abandon every preventative technique such as checking, testing, watching for the warning signs of the top ten illnesses? Not if that approach suits your needs. We are saying that if we want a positive result *in* our health, we must think totally positive *about* our health. And there is no exception to that rule.

Has there ever been a day when a newspaper headline read, "The Health Flu sweeps the Nation?" No! Or a time when a health expert on the six o'clock news described all the warning signs of "Radiant Health"? How about a new statistic on the cover of a health magazine that said, "Energy, Ease and Exuberance expected to hit 9 out of 10 people this year!" Sounds absurd? Unfortunately, it is. As far as headlines, newscasts and magazine covers, the *positive* focus is on *negative* effects. Sadly, the final results support the initial focus.

With the help of the media

The point of society's positive focus on negative results is well proven with an exercise in our workshop. We distribute 'health' articles from newspapers, magazines and brochures. Each table of people gets 10 - 15 different articles on topics ranging from "Spiritual Healing" to the "Mounting statistics of those with heart disease." Everyone is asked to choose an article that typifies the health education that they are used to seeing in the media. 80 - 90% of the people choose an article that vividly explains the warning signs, statistics or manifestations of some illness. A small percentage choose an article on stress management or nutrition. Once in awhile someone chooses an article on the wondrous healing power within.

The point of this exercise is to show that everywhere we look, the graphic details of what could go wrong with our health, blaze the headlines. It is no secret that articles on disasters sell lots of newspapers, but the media is also one of our most powerful sources of suggestion. Every product that we buy from cat food to computers is determined by the media. Can we see now that when the media broadcasts illness after illness, warning after warning, it only helps to spread the bad news throughout our minds and our bodies? Whether selling product or panic; news flashes on TV, broadcasts on the radio, detailed brochures with full color pictures, if the media is selling, America is buying. When it comes to being sold on the graphic details of what could go wrong with the body, it behooves us as intelligent, logical beings to muster a strong dose of sales resistance.

Although we are certainly seeing the 'lifesaving' logic of focusing on the positive side of health versus the negative side of illness, seeing actual results will take some time. At this point, *awareness* is all

that is expected. Staying open to the possibility that we have a
power on the inside that far supercedes any problem on the outside,
is the first step in discovering 'health beyond *belief*.' Just awakening to the mania about every ill that could happen will help us think
twice before buying all this 'B.S.' from now on. But customer, be-
ware, business is business. As long as there are products to sell,
there will be powerful salespeople and highly creative sales pitches.
And health or rather *disease* is no exception to this rule. Health, or
rather *disease* is a multibillion dollar sales industry. We are brought
up to believe that pharmaceuticals (legal drugs), and doctors are or-
dained by God. Rarely do we think that they need to meet sales
quotas like any other business. We would like to meet personally
the geniuses of the advertising agencies who are behind the big
drug companies campaigns. Who else but a genius could sell the
entire American public on the idea that health, an energy more
powerful than electricity, could be bought in a pill? As we said
loud and clear earlier, anything couched with the 'fear of death' is a
highly effective selling technique. When we focus on fear,
(especially fear of dying), it blinds our sense of logic. But when we
focus on logic, it obliterates fear. Logic, rather than fear, is a far
healthier focus.

What are we teaching our kids today?

To see how the focus on sickness (in the guise of 'health' can have
disastrous results, all we need to do is check out any public school
system. The accepted belief is that every school system is a *hotbed
of illness*, where sickness is spread through the school from one
student to another until half the student body is down with the flu.
We have had the opportunity to work with many school systems
and found evidence to suggest a far subtler culprit. Working with
students on this idea of positive thinking, we are pleased that
schools are beginning to accept the value of the mind. But the acceptance is short-lived, school systems, like the rest of society make
a disastrous exception when it comes to health. School nurse's

office are decorated with all the latest ills. From articles on 'flu season' to vivid photographs of a deadly virus, walking in there is
enough to make anyone sick. It is positive all right, positive that
students will come down with something before the semester ends.
Talking with many of these nurses, (who ironically are 'out sick'
quite often themselves), have revealed a most interesting pattern.
The occurrence of student illness rises every year, and most of
these students have already diagnosed themselves before walking
into the office. From all they have heard, read and seen, especially
in their own school nurses office, these students have a fairly good
idea of the ill from which they suffer. Have these students really
'caught' something or are they just caught in the web of sickness
suggestion? Logic and experience definitely point to the latter.

Sickness; no longer shocking to the senses

The focus in our society on health *problems* instead of healing *power*, has gotten out of hand. Every year more and more is added to
the list of what could go wrong with our body. Whether a brand
new ill, or just a new hybrid of an old ill, our society has become
obsessed with illness. Is this supposed to represent a healthy state
of mind? What is most disconcerting is that the barrage of ills is so
common to our eyes, ears and minds that we have become immune
to the noise. While the sick talk may not *consciously* hit us anymore, *subconsciously,* we absorb every word and the media banks
on this. But if we are not yet shocked at the blaze of negativity surrounding our Health Care System, let's take another look at how
'health' is promoted. With new eyes and ears, look closely at the
magazine articles that talk about 'health.' Also listen to the news
broadcasts that feature a 'health' report. Finally, eavesdrop on any
conversation between two or more people discussing their version
of 'health;' they occur in almost anyplace, at almost anytime. It is
time that we conduct our own 'health study'. We will be shocked at
how many of these articles, newscasts and conversations focus on
pain and illness. Even if it is in a preventative way, focus is focus.

Hearing about pain and illness for the purpose of preventing them does not take away the disastrous effects, no matter how much we have been lead to believe otherwise. We may have become immune to hearing about pain and illness but we *cannot* become immune to the resulting negative effects. As is the case with any idea that our mind focuses on, the outer life follows like an obedient servant. Are we finally beginning to accept the fact that health is no longer the exception to this rule?

The path of pathology

So how does our traditional Health Care System lead us on this misguided path of pathology? It gives us positive landmarks to verify the track that we are on. With each health problem, from a simple cold to a serious ill, landmarks or warning signs have been created to guide us along the path of pathology. "Your throat will be scratchy, eyes watery, nose running." This so called preventative approach, focusing on the warning signs of every ill imaginable, is likely to be creating and recreating the problem. We have been led to believe that early detection is *preventative*. Looking for, expecting or focusing on anything, warning sign or not, is *creative* not preventative. The proven principle of, "What a person can conceive and believe, they can achieve," does not have an addendum that says, "except in health." Whatever a person conceives and believes from the symptoms of success to the symptoms of the flu, the mind being no respecter of purpose, will work to make the objective of focus a reality.

If filling the mind with all the signs of impending sickness doesn't become fatal, it certainly kills all hope of radiant health. As for the person who has viewed their frequent urination as the first sign of disaster, the endless fear can be just as bad as the impending illness. We have been friends with Laurie for many years and have watched what learned panic can do to a creative, healthy woman. Since a child, she has been convinced that she was 'dying' of something. Although we joke, "You can't have a brain tumor, we're going down the shore this weekend," it is very obvious that the worry is killing her. There is no doubt that the mental branding of the 'warning signs' has contributed greatly to her fear of illness. Working for many years in the traditional health care field, Laurie has studied medical journals and fact sheets on many of the most dreaded ills. Unknowingly she has so memorized and visualized the many symptoms and signs, that even slight dizziness or a little bit of tingling in her hands sends Laurie into a panic. She says that her mind is getting the best of her, but deep in her heart, the fear echoes day and night. As the symptoms die down and she realizes she is not dying, the panic subsides. But Laurie's fears are always bubbling at the surface just waiting for another sign to appear which given a few months always do.

No one knows whether Laurie's vivid pictures of what could go wrong with her body, set in place by a mindful list of warning signs, will actually create the ill some day. We are helping her to dispel that possibility. In a way with this fear, she is dying a little each day in spirit. The days weeks and years of fears, draining the life out of her, always putting a dark cloud over any happiness that she may have is no way to live. No one should live with the fear of death or disaster popping up everytime they scratch their head, (a new warning sign?). Unfortunately anyone who is not caught in this web of warning signs is the exception to the rule. Most of us do not consciously panic like Laurie does, but even a common cold is often created by focusing on the 'early warning signs.' What comes to mind when we sneeze a few extra times, feel our throat scratchy or experience a wave of fatigue? We probably think, "Oh, I'm getting a cold!" and lo and behold, within minutes or hours, we are right! The key question here is, are we being *intuitive* or *creative?* If this were about our career and we noticed some sign of problems, the successful and smart thing would be to take the problems in stride, avoid focusing on failure, and continue to create and visualize the outcome being successful. Yes, we would all agree on that approach as the wise thing to do. But when it comes to health, as far as the rules of positive thinking, all bets are off. Heed the warning signs, prepare for the worst, keep checking for the outcome that we *don't* want, read up on the impending ill and visit every specialist on the condition. Something is *fatally* wrong with this picture!

Finally in the 'market' for health

About 10 years ago when we were just realizing this 'wolf in sheep's clothing, (illness masked as health), we created our famous *7 Warning Signs of Health* poster. We had become painfully aware that for every ill from a cold to a cancer, migraines to heart disease, there was a list of warning signs. To most people at that time, being constantly reminded to look for the current signs of a future ill was not only normal, it was considered the wise approach to health. Knowing our God given right to health and using the principle of logic, we felt quite strongly otherwise. The conviction to do something about this focus on problems hit us while food shopping one day. On the grocery bags, catching everyone's conscious or subconscious eye, was a list of "the 7 Warning Signs" of a most dreaded disease. Talk about shopping for sickness! Shocked and determined to finally give the other side of this picture, we created a list of "the 7 Warning Signs" of impending, radiant health. These signs like those of almost every major illness, were natural and normal functions of the body and mind. Only this time, different than with those of disease, these natural, normal symptoms were *positive*. They were the 'warning signs' of and the steps to physical, mental and spiritual health. The 'warning signs' of health, what a concept! The poster is our 'trademark' and they've been seen and ordered from around the country. These posters are featured in true health magazines and are in the possession of Dr. Bernie Siegel, Og Mandino, Dr. Deepak Chopra, Dr. Wayne Dyer, and Dr. Bob Owen, some of the incredible holistic and spiritual teachers whose writings have been such a part of our inspiration.

The 7 Warning Sign of Health poster was intended to make a positive and strong statement. We were clear about the reason the poster was created and why it was needed. If a person wanted health, from bright, clear eyes to a oneness with God (warning signs 1 and 7), they would have to study health, focus on health and look for health. It is just a matter of logic.

Who would have thought that this concept, "A Negative Approach to Positive Thinking," would have had such far reaching effects. Even though as a society, we are sold on the truth that positive thinking is our most powerful birthright, it was shown in this chapter that health is taken as the rightful exception to this rule! The first proof of this was when we discussed how anger and fear are the subtle tools used to keep us bound and gagged to the traditional health system. Quite a negative approach right up front. But the negativity went deeper. It doesn't take a brain surgeon to realize that focusing on pain, chronic health problems and serious disease is never going to create health. If we follow the rules of logic, positive thinking or the principle of "As you sow, sow shall you reap," then whatever we focus on, positive or negative, is never preventative, but always *creative*. We have to ask ourselves, "What am I really creating for my health?"

Labels. . . are they putting our health in jeopardy?

In our health workshops, group exercises work well to get everyone personally involved and most importantly to drive home the point of how deep the 'B.S.' in health really is. Health Jeopardy is one of our favorite exercises because it is quick, humorous and proves two major points in one. The purpose is to see how quickly, given one clue and the first letter of the word, a person can access their vast knowledge of 'health' labels. Let's see how many we can get 'right'.

(1)   The label for a severe headache starting with 'M'.
       What is _____ ?

(2)   The label for stiff joints starting with 'A'.
       What is _____ ?

(3)   The label for a curved spine starting with 'S'.
       What is _____ ?

(4)   The two word label for severe fatigue starting with 'E'.
       What is _____ ?

(5)   The label for great difficulty in breathing starting with
       an 'A.' What is _____?

(6)   The label for a severe cold in the lungs starting with a
       'P.' What is _____?

(7)   The two word label for a common allergy starting with
       'H'. What is _____?

(8)   The label for a hole in the stomach lining starting with
       'U'. What is _____?

(9)   The three word label that causes difficulty using the
       wrist starting with 'C'. What is _____?

(10)   The label for chronic high blood pressure starting with
       an 'H'. What is _____?

*(Answers: (1) Migraine, (2) Arthritis, (3) Scoliosis, (4) Epstein Barr, (5)
Asthma, (6) Pneumonia, (7) Hay Fever, (8) Ulcer, (9) Carpel Tunnel
Syndrome, (10) Hypertension.)*

There are actually twenty labels to name in this exercise and almost everyone in the audience gets at least seventeen right, usually within two seconds of the clue. Judging by the smiles on their faces, participants in this game feel smart and quite proud of their vast 'health' knowledge. We explain that the purpose of this exercise was not to measure how clever we are, but rather how *conditioned*. This may have just been a game of Jeopardy, but having immediate access to the medical term for every ill from AIDS to Z is putting our health in *jeopardy*! We have become so familiar with health or rather *illness* labels that given one simple clue, we can make a sophisticated diagnosis for ourselves and everyone around us. Contrary to popular opinion, this knowledge makes us stuck not smart. Going back to the principle of positive thinking, any idea that we focus on or know like the back of our hand, is creative to our body. And the worst part is that labels have no 'statute of limitations', they are too often with us for life. "Once an allergy sufferer, always an allergy sufferer." Keep a label in the mind long enough and it becomes us, or we become it. How many people do we know, if not ourselves that have become associated with a rather 'sick' label. "I have arthritis." "I am an asthmatic." "There goes my hay fever, again." We know the danger of negative labels in all other areas of life. Labeling someone stupid, unattractive, unlovable or a failure can disable a person for life. How can we possible consider illness labels as an exception to this rule?

There is another handicap to being illness smart and label wise. If a simple clue can bring up the name of an illness in two seconds, what might a *symptom* do? How quickly does a label rush to the surface of our mind and panic rush to the chambers of our heart when any unusual physical symptom appears? We have been warned to stay so 'in tune' with our body, (could we practice that idea on our mind?), that a natural healing or a process that seems unnatural to us, sends our brains into overdrive. "What does this mean?" "I read about this." "I'll bet I'm coming down with. . ."

Dr. Michael Fitzgerald, a wholistic chiropractor and dear friend knows full well the harm that a label can do. Over the years that our families have been working with Dr. Mike, he could have diagnosed a whole slew of labels for the many symptoms that we have had. Previous to going to him, many medical doctors had done just that, causing what could have been a temporary ill to last for weeks, months or years. Dr. Mike has never given us a label, instead he explains the problem in terms of a zone in the body that is malfunctioning, (as taught by the teachings of the founder of Concept-Therapy, Dr. Thurman Fleet.)[1] He always suggests that the zone will be back to normal in no time, (positive thinking used correctly.) This suggestion along with but not dependent upon, a chiropractic adjustment and the chance to express or release our feelings, always relieves the symptoms and heals the problem. Is Dr. Mike a miracle worker? Not really. He just knows the laws of the mind, particularly regarding the effects of labels, and therefore never illicits fear in the minds of his patients with negative labels. He has implicit faith in the healing power within each patient and knows without a doubt that if a patient will open to this power and then live the laws of health (not the laws of disease), they will be well.

The last but certainly not the least problem with labels is the *prestige* that they instill. Some people take offense when we suggest that labels instill a sense of self importance. Many people that we have talked with over the years have felt special after being given a sophisticated name for their ill. The reason that we can venture such a claim, having been guilty ourselves is because of the endless stories that we hear. Like the 'big fish' story where the fish gets bigger everytime the story is told, labels also get bigger everytime their story is told. We have heard so many people discuss the label that they were given with such enthusiasm and repetition to anyone who will listen, that we can only come to one conclusion; some people *like* being 'ill' labeled. Whether a person happens to be the first on their block with a particular ill, or on the other side, they

---

[1]   Concept-Therapy Institute and Courses, 25550 Boerne Stage Rd, San Antonio, TX, 78255, 1-800-531-5628

have 'joined the club', a label bestows a special kind of attention on the recipient. Sometimes they help us form a sense of camaraderie. On the TV Show, "thirty something" back in the late '80's, one of the main characters was trying to *bond* with another person during a dinner party. Frantically looking for something in common to connect them, she shouted excitedly, "You have a bleeding ulcer? Wow! So do I!" What a way to feel connected.

Labels; these so called reality checks have become the foundation of our life, especially with health. We may have been led to believe that they *define* our condition, but can we now see how they really *confine* it? While labels may help us to feel grounded and secure, (we like knowing who we are and where we are headed) they can make it impossible to break free of the condition. Dr. Deepak Chopra, a respected holistic doctor and author, confirms the limits of labels. Dr. Chopra, in his book "Ageless Body, Timeless Mind," says (and we paraphrase), that although we in the scientific community have raised the possible life span in our society from 75 to 120 years, appearing to be quite an improved standard, we still have limited the possibilities. By doing this, the age of 120 will form the ceiling to which, if we believe the label, will never be exceeded, if ever reached. Pat practiced this de-labeling idea with her cat, Samantha, who was still catching birds and mice at 20 years old with no claws! She died at 22 years young!

In the last few decades, the effects of labels on children have become widely studied. Label a child, even just with our own *thoughts*, as lazy, academically slow, a troublemaker or unlikely to amount to anything, reinforce it over time, and it will take the strength of Samson for the child to break this mold. A parent or teacher without an understanding of the power of suggestion will think themselves intuitive when the child manifests the previously diagnosed label. "I just knew they would be trouble." "I was right, this kid has no head for math." "I just knew that you would be a sickly kid."

Starting from conception, it has been shown that children respond
to the thoughts, voice and feelings of their mom and dad. They are
therefore, susceptible to negative influences much more easily. We
need to use our heads and think before we label a child's fertile
mind for life with an idea that we *don't* want expressed. Well
meaning parents, family members and teachers must realize the importance of negative labeling. Talking to or even thinking about a
child with a sick *sense* makes them more susceptible to a chronic
health problem than any germs could.

If you asked one hundred people to categorize themselves name,
professional status and chronic ill, the last would flow as easily as
the first. Literally thousands of labels have been created for every
ill imaginable. What makes them so dangerous is that they are now
in medical terms, instead of human terms. These labels are far less
personal and far more clinical which makes them far too complicated to heal easily. Labels, like migraines, have complicated the
idea of headaches. Epstein Barr doesn't sound at all like exhaustion. Arthritis is far removed from stiff joints. Dare we think
that these rather sophisticated labels are *meant* to confuse and over-
whelm us? Could there be a gain to the Health Care System if we
are at a loss to understand our own ills? Maybe we would be wiser
to *call them as we see them*, to call our pain or problem in simple
terms that even a child could understand. It may sound rather foolish to use terms like *bellyache*, my *head hurts*, or *boo-boo*, but if
like children, we heal quickly, whose the fool?

Maybe negative labeling works well in the area of addictions. A
person with a serious alcohol or drug problem may need to constantly remind themselves of their addiction in order to stay clean.
This attachment to the problem obviously has its negative side.
When, if ever, are we no longer 'an alcoholic'? By the same token,
when, if ever, are we no longer 'an arthritic'? Which comes first,
the healing of the label or the healing of the body? According to all
the creative principles of life, from positive thinking to 'As you sow,

you reap', it must be the label. And since we now have over 3,000 labels of illnesses, we have some serious healing to do.

So, should all labels be eliminated from our health system? No, just the sick ones. Healthy labels like 'strong immune system'. . . 'bright, clear eyes'. . . 'energy and exuberance'. . . should be branded on ourselves and everyone we love in thought as well as word.

Never say die

A very famous philosopher back in the 1950's (before Alternative Health was even an alternative), went to visit a very sick friend. He knew that his friend had been diagnosed (which means 'I guess'), as seriously ill. Upon walking into his hospital room, instead of the usual, "So, how are you feeling?" and "What did the doctors say?", this philosopher turned the whole sick scene around. With a smile and a truly caring heart, he said to his friend, "So good to see you, you look radiant." With a puzzled look, the friend said, "Didn't they tell you what I've got?" The philosopher still smiling said, "No, and I don't care to know. I see you as radiantly well. And while we are on the subject, you should do the same. Keep the ill in your body if you must, but for God's sake, get it out of your mind!" Well, the friend did just that. He cut the ill out of his thoughts and to his surprise as well as his doctors, the friend recovered quickly. This story was told to educate us on the power of thoughts and words. They have the potential to fill a person with healing hope. They also have the potential to kill all hope as in the case with our friend Derrick.

Derrick went for a routine physical in the middle of October several years back. After filling his heart with dread, putting him through test after test, the doctors finally 'found' what they labeled to be leukemia. Within a few days, this vivacious, funny, high spirited guy was in a hospital bed given six weeks to live. Well, the doctors were right on the money; he died before the New Year. What really cut his life down to nothing? Was it the label leukemia which automatically comes with the image of incurable, or was it the actual disease? The truth will never be known except to our late friend and God. But the question must be asked. Only through logic of how the mind and body work together coupled with the experience of seeing its effects in our life will the truth come to us.

If we ever want to be free of the ill we must first be free of its label. If we ever hope to experience our heritage of radiant health, we must first create a label for it. The "I am radiantly healthy" label may need to come first before we actually see it in our body. This is nothing but *logic*. But in our complicated, impersonal, impossible to understand medical jargon, could this idea of a real health label be too simple to be accepted as truth?

There is so much 'B.S.' surrounding 'B.S.' # 1: Health is the exception to the rule, but the power of our own logic can melt away much of it, and soon our experience will verify it. Breaking any limiting belief system occurs when the 'B.S.' can no longer pass the test of logic. Health being the exception to the rules of life is quickly failing that test.

2. Personal and Spiritual Power

Using logic and the principle Positive Thinking or as *we* call it, a 'Negative Approach to Positive Thinking,' it was shown how society has made health the exception to the rule that works in all other areas of life. But as was also clearly shown, positive is positive and negative is negative; no matter what the original purpose, preventative included, there are no exceptions to this rule. There are two more principles that fall under *the exception to the rule* 'B.S.' The next one is the principle of Personal and Spiritual power. Our society has taken another potent principle and tried to hide it when it comes to health. Through the lack of understanding on this principle, we as a society have put self imposed limits on our unlimited power. Socrates, Jesus, Emerson, Einstein and hundreds of others have proven that there is an unlimited creative power within us.

This awesome power responds to our grandest wish as well as our least inclination. That is the good news. The bad news is that many of our least inclinations, (belief systems), are killing us! Fearing a major illness, focusing on our headaches or labeling ourselves with a reoccurring condition, although mostly on a subconscious level inclines the creative power within us toward that state. With such a magnitude of power within us ready to respond to our suggestions - 'B.S.' or not - we must refrain from consciously or unconsciously concentrating on illness.

The rampant stress, sadness and sickness viewed as 'normal' in this world is the price that we have paid for ignoring our own inner power. Logically speaking, there is only one solution. The ease of our stress, the answer to our sadness and yes, the healing of our sickness, all lies in one source; the divine power within. God knows we have tried looking everywhere else, but until we make our life's purpose to become one with this power, all attempts at peace, happiness and yes, health will be lost. Thankfully, we have a New Age movement, (it is really an "Old Age" revisited.) In the last fifteen years, there has been a deluge of books and tape on the power within. Although the knowledge has been around for thousands of years, *using* it in everyday life is brand new. But the times, they are a-changin.

Two thousand years ago, Jesus, the most spiritually connected of our philosophers gave us two life saving principles, "As a man thinketh in his heart, so is he," and "If ye have faith as a grain of mustard seed, ye shall say unto the mountain, 'remove hence to yonder place', and it shall remove and nothing shall be impossible to you." Did he footnote those two principles with the line, "in all areas of life *except* in health." On the contrary, Jesus added, "and all these things I can do, you can do even greater." If one of the greatest minds of all time proclaimed that we have the 'power to move mountains,' how come when it comes to health, even the little molehills seem to have power over us? The reason is simple. We are taught that health, unlike any other area of life is something to be *feared* instead of *freed.* Thanks to the promotion of panic in our society, (we would rather vaccinate than educate), health and illness seem to be immune to the truths of the ages. Biblical prophecies like, "Whatsoever ye desire, ask and ye shall receive," seem to become impotent when it comes to health. Even though the world is slow to change, for those who incorporate it into their Health Plan, and have faith in the healing power within, even if only as big as a mustard seed, "nothing shall be impossible."

Doreen remembers vividly using this 'mustard seed' principle to heal her intense fears during the birth of her daughter. After almost 24 hours of labor, she was only five centimeters dilated. (She needed to get to ten centimeters before pushing the baby out). The doctor said that the baby was quite big and worse, probably stuck. He then said a Cesarean was most likely the only solution. Even at the brink of collapse, Doreen set her mind away from the result. Right or wrong, she had said from the beginning that she would deliver her child vaginally. But time was almost up, (and her 'B.S.' that she waits till the last minute in almost everything was automatically operating) her mountain of a child still hadn't budged. Doreen's brother, along with the rest of her family were waiting in the lounge. Upon hearing the forecast, he ran to his car and got his Rays of the Dawn[2] book, (first book every written by Dr. Fleet). When he gave it to Doreen, without thinking or looking, she opened right up to Jesus' famous principle, "If ye have faith as a grain of mustard seed, ye can say unto the mountain, 'remove hence to yonder place' and it shall remove and nothing shall be impossible to you." Doreen remembers feeling a surge of energy running through her totally exhausted body and with what seemed like no time, her little 'mountain' moved and she dilated to ten centimeters. The doctor was in shock. He said later that he never would have believed the baby could move so much, so quickly. He obviously didn't know Jesus' prophecy and he definitely didn't know Doreen's will!

---

[2] The Rays of the Dawn, Concept-Therapy Institute, 25550 Boerne Stage Rd., San Antonio, TX.78255, 1-800-531-5628

Judging from the way that the marketing of Health Care is going, it may take another millennium before society as a whole becomes immune to its mind grabbing campaigns. But as was the case in the movie "The Poseidon Adventure," we don't have to wait for the ship to sink to realize that the masses were wrong. Our unlimited power does not need to wait for the support of the world when it has always had the support of the universe.

3. The Right to Think, Question and Disagree

Can we still accept the 'B.S.' that the power that *made* the body and *sustains* the body is incompetent to *heal* the body? Is losing touch with our unlimited source of healing the negative side effect of our drug obsessed Health Care System? Thank God we live in a society where we have the right to ask the questions. . . or do we? There is an unwritten law suggesting that non health professionals - you and I - should defer most, if not all, of their health decisions to the 'experts'.

We in America pride ourselves on analyzing, researching and differing with expert opinion. We believe that our feelings, intuition and sense of logic are highly valuable in every area of life. Why then when it comes to our health, do we accept almost everyone else's ideas over our own? Anyone from a doctor to the doorman can sway or scare us with the latest 'health' bulletin. "Studies with rats proved that broccoli prevents psoriasis." Nail polish may cause cancer. (Does that mean darker shades are more potent?) A few strong words from just about anyone and another theory is concocted. How many of them are really 'breakthroughs' and how many are just more 'B.S.' ? The cartoon character "Ziggy" best answered that question. While watching the six o'clock news, Ziggy was intrigued by the latest health warning. It said, "Everything that was *good* for you last year is now *bad,* and vice versa!" The wisdom of wit.

Thinking, questioning and disagreeing with traditional health practices may put a person in a healthier position but also a precarious
one. Few people even if they feel right in their hearts, are free from
the good opinions of others, with disapproval and rejection being a
'fate worse than death.' But for those of us who are ready for a
wholistic approach to health, this fate will no doubt be faced. Time
and again, we have heard about well meaning friends and relatives
who get quite indignant at 'alternative health' practices, even if they
are working better than the traditional methods! A client of ours
summarized the whole situation best. After hearing the ranting and
raving from her in-laws about her choice for a more natural approach to healing, she shook her head and said, "You would think
they had stock in the drug companies!" These well meaning people
might be subtly doubting their own methods and worried about
their future health. Fear is often the precursor to anger and criticism. We may never change *them*, all we can do is strengthen *us*.

One of the most limiting but at the same time universally accepted
beliefs is that a 'doctor' knows more about our health than we do.
But *think* about that for a moment, is that really logical? Who
could possibly know our physical, mental and spiritual needs *better*
than *we* do. Given a 10 - 20 minute visit every once in a while, how
well can they really know us, not just our body, but the *whole* of
us? Looking at this twisted logic another way, would we allow an
outsider to determine our potential for great success? Unless they
lived inside our being, their determination would be biased at best,
and completely wrong at worst. Why then do we assume that an
outsider can determine our potential for health? Even the most
learned of health experts are at a disadvantage when it comes to *our*
health. No one has the intimate connection with our feelings, our
needs and our intuitive guidance that we have, we are with us 24
hours a day! And it is within such feelings, needs and intuitive
guidance that all the answers to our healing lie. (This will be further explained in the coming chapters). Does that mean that we
should ignore everyone else's opinions? Not necessarily. A supportive, positive *health partner* is just what the doctor ordered.

Such a partner can be a book, a tape, a talk with God or a discussion with the physician of our persuasion. In the process of partnering, however, our needs, feelings and intuition must be held in the highest light. They are contrary to past belief, of truly *expert* opinion.

Americans are known for many things, but taking things quietly sitting down and without an opinion is not one of them. We live in a society where *freedom of speech* is practiced for all its worth. We in the good old U.S.A. are free to voice our opinion, especially concerning our own life, and do just that at every opportunity. So why when it comes to the 'God of Medicine' do we become as quiet as a church mouse? We have no problem *thinking, questioning and disagreeing* with everything from politics to pollution. But when it comes to health, *our* health, we forget to think, are afraid to question and wouldn't dare disagree.

Whether we forfeit our right to think, question and disagree with health professionals because we are afraid of being sick or afraid of being disapproved of, (or both), fear is the real 'health problem'. And faith, faith in our own inner guidance as well as our own inner healer, is the only solution to the health problem. Just because this approach to health doesn't yet conform to the norm shouldn't discourage us from learning all we can about it. Fortunately, more and more people are 'into' alternatives. And people don't mind being 'different' as long as there are plenty of others who are different in the same way!

The health monopoly

Putting the best interests of the American public at the forefront, our society has all but done away with every form of monopoly in business. Obviously the reason that divestiture is encouraged in American enterprise is (a) it prevents any one industry from getting so powerful that it *controls* its customers, and (b) it allows growth in the industry and healthy competition, so that the service or product is constantly being improved. The threat of customer control, as well as the choice of bigger profits over product refinement is the occupational hazard of any monopoly. And one of the largest monopolies, the American health industry, is no exception to this rule.

It isn't easy to *think, question or disagree* with any authority, but a monopoly as large as the American health industry makes it even harder. Up until quite recently, if we got thrown out of the Health Care System, we would have no where to go. Fortunately, there are more and more alternatives to this 'medical monopoly'; thinking, questioning and disagreeing to name a few. The silent suggestion of *think at your own risk,* keeps us as a society enslaved to a fearful and sick approach to health. The truth is that *not thinking,* not using our divine wisdom and logic puts us at the greatest risk. In our own personal experience, it is just this type of approach, *logically and divinely thinking for ourselves* that has taken the dread and hopelessness out of our idea of health. We are no longer intimidated by someone with a 'health degree'. We look instead for those who have a healthy degree of insight, who understand the inner workings of our outer health. Even then, we form a partnership, not a doctatorship.

But this 'having a mind of our own' must be rightfully earned to lead to radiant health. Indiscriminate resistance just to exert our own will is only the other side of this sick approach to health. Thinking for ourselves must not be a scapegoat for a rebellious nature. Fighting purely to vent anger is just as 'sick' as totally suppressing our feelings (we know it well, it's how we began). The point is to look at our blinding 'B.S.', eliminate that which cannot stand the test of logic and then grow with the higher principles of healing. This is a lifetime process. With that kind of clear minded thinking along with the assistance of true 'health' experts, we become qualified to diagnose our own needs, health no longer being the exception to this rule. By the way, since we as a society have become so big on 'second opinions,' wouldn't it be of the highest wisdom for that second opinion to be our own?

Health. . . no longer the exception to the rule

We can debate why until we turn blue, but the fact remains that our society takes quite an exception to the creative process of life when it comes to health. It may be subtle but this first Belief System is more damaging to our present and future potential of health than all the 'B.S.' on earth. This belief is also the most stubborn. The idea that illness is just a natural part of life, that with the exception of a miracle, we are powerless to change, is pounded into our heads every time we open a newspaper. That kind of fear can paralyze even the most *positive* of thinkers. Living with the dread of disease slowly sapping our strength until *if* and *when* a cure for all ills is found is no way to live; neither is living with the fear of financial failure until *if* and *when* we win the lottery. Both scenarios render our natural human potential, our unlimited creative power within, impotent. Why anxiously *wait* for miracles when we were born with the power to *create* them?

The purpose of this book is (1) to eliminate the dread and despair that looms over our heads about illness and (2) to create within our being a path through which radiant health can naturally flow. In order to attain to such a state of joy and freedom we must first awaken to the truth about health. The first truth is that we are loaded down with 'B.S.' This 'B.S.' is the first order of healing. Secondly, we must realize that the principles of *Positive Thinking* and *Personal or Spiritual Power* are just as potent with health as they are with any other area of life. With those principles back in business as far as our health is concerned, we have the right and the wisdom to *Think, Question and Disagree* when appropriate. It is all just a matter of logic, pure powerful logic.

'B.S.' # 2:
Our Health Care System
can and *should* take responsibility
for our Health

Maybe we assume too much. Given society's mounting fears of serious illness, the rise in headaches, backaches, allergies, and all other chronic problems, not to mention the outrageous insurance costs, we automatically figured that health was the most pressing issue on everyone's mind. We also took for granted that each person would be willing to do whatever it takes to get and stay healthy. We assumed too much. For reasons that we are about to discuss in this section, unless the health plan were quick, practically effortless and preferably in the form of a pill, doing whatever it takes, often came down to doing as *little* as it takes.

Jay, a client, had been complaining for some time about constant headaches. He had been to several doctors, gotten some pills, but the pain persisted making him wonder if it could be something 'serious.' While talking on the phone one evening to Doreen, Jay said that he had read about what persistent headaches might be leading to and the prognosis left him scared to death every time his head throbbed. It was obvious that he was sick and tired of the pain, the pills that didn't work and the fatal fears that hounded him every day. Sounding desperate for a solution, Jay seemed willing to do whatever it took (so we thought), to heal the problem. Doreen and Jay talked about how the crux of our pain and ills was not because of a limited healing *ability* but rather a limited healing *approach.* They discussed how all of us have a power running *through* us that is far greater than any problem that comes *to* us. Knowing Jay's faith in positive thinking, Doreen spent time explaining how our health system has taken a negative approach to positive thinking. She explained that this focus, almost totally on the problem, tells us to check for the warning signs of every terminal illness possible and then dispenses labels like migraines, brain tumors and cancer as quickly as they dispense pills. She also explained that filling our minds with all the serious indications of headaches is negative, not preventative. Seeing the vision of what we want, she went on to explain, and then expecting *that* outcome is the best 'health insurance' we can have.

After ten minutes it seemed a good time to get to the core of the problem. Doreen asked Jay if his *outer* headaches could in any way reflect his *inner* headaches; could he be feeling overburdened, worried that everything was on his *head?* It was a rhetorical question. Jay, like many in our 'stress for success' society was deeply troubled by life in general, making a good living, specifically. His unrelenting throbbing head reflected his unrelenting throbbing worry and guilt, an obvious example of the mind/body connection. If he released the inner headaches (the worry and guilt), the healing power would then be free to flow to his outer headaches. The healing power knows no limits except the ones we give it.

After the talk, Jay did seem less panicky and very grateful. Maybe this was a sign that he was ready to do whatever it took to regain his health. After giving him lists of books and audio tapes to help him create this new level of health, it was suggested that he take the next Concept-Therapy seminar available. In a solemn voice, Jay asked if he could call back later. Thinking that he needed some time to absorb all this new information, Doreen said "I guess you have a lot to think about," "No," he said quite innocently, "it's 7:30 and I don't want to miss the Simpson's."

Being upstaged by a cartoon sitcom will stop anyone in their tracks. It made us realize that not everyone is ready or willing to do what it takes to be truly healthy.

There is no question that our society *needs* this wholistic ideal of health, but that doesn't mean that they *want* it; want to do what it takes, that is. It is not that much different with any other area of life. Millions of people in our society need more money, but far less are willing to do all that it takes to earn more. The same applies to physical fitness, weight loss, relationships and spiritual growth. Almost everyone would gladly accept a leaner body, a more loving relationship and a closer connection to God, but how many are willing to trade their scheduled time in front of the TV to get there?

For those who have learned or instinctively know that health is not a *curative* but rather a *creative* process, that it cannot be obtained through someone or something else, that it must be primarily *created* from within, this book will be a blessing. It is for those who are sick and tired of the aches, pains and fears of life threatening illness. It is also for those who want to experience the upper limits of radiant health and are willing to do whatever it takes to get there. We lose more people on that last condition. That is where we lost Jay.

Tom, another client, also bailed out at this point of doing whatever it takes. Tom had what the doctors called a very 'serious' condition. Over the last ten years he had two heart bypass operations, had developed diabetes and although clinically alive, felt like he was slowly dying. A man who just a few years ago was strong as an ox, was now having trouble walking half a block. Breathing had become a major effort and his once powerful legs had swollen so much that just standing was very painful. Tom was the type of person that you didn't ask how he was feeling, because he would tell you. After hearing all the gory details about the pain, the medications, the current prognosis, the weekly doctor visits, the expected surgeries, you would walk away queasy yourself.

If you asked Tom about life before the ills, he would say how much he loved to work outdoors, couldn't wait to get up at four in the morning to go fishing and dreamed about traveling the world. The brightness returned to Tom's face when he talked about the 'good old days.' During those 'good old days', he only needed four or five hours sleep a night and was up like a rocket each day. Tom says that now all he *does* is sleep.

After we asked Tom about any major impact that occurred in his life right before the symptoms appeared, he said with tears in his eyes that he had lost his oldest daughter during that time. She had been killed in a car accident. What made it unbearable was that Tom argued with her right before she died. Losing his daughter was tragic, but the guilt over arguing with her right before almost killed *him*, he said. We can all relate to this story because all of us have unresolved guilt, guilt over situations that are nowhere near as tragic as this one. Was it just a coincidence that Tom had said that the guilt almost killed him and within a short time he had developed a *physical condition* that almost killed him? Was it also a coincidence that this grief over a kind of lost love should hit his heart?

Was there any way to help ease Tom's pain? From all we'd learned and experienced ourselves the only way to heal his heart was through self forgiveness and letting go. But would these words of wisdom really make any sense? Where in all our advanced academic education did a course on forgiveness; surrendering to the path of inner peace ever come up? Where, except through some misunderstood cliché, have we been taught that everything happens for a reason, a good reason? Yes, these truths are the 'cure' for most, if not all of our ills, but how do we bridge the gap between these ideals and real life? Each time Tom spoke of his emotional or physical pain, we strongly suggested alternative health practices that have had much success with conditions like his. Books and tapes on healing and forgiveness are suggested, along with going to Dr. Mike and a course in Concept-Therapy. Tom's reactions were much like those of Jay. He would listen politely then excuse himself for lunch, a doctors appointment, or his midday medication.

Tom showed disgust over his all consuming ills, but what he never showed was a true willingness to change. Was it really easier to go for another triple bypass than to change a single belief? We don't believe that his reluctance to change was because he enjoyed the pain, the drugs or the constant fear of dying. From what he had been told by the well meaning medical society, who could blame him for his less than enthusiastic attitude? He was given such little hope of ever living a normal life and a prognosis that he would slowly deteriorate over time. With that kind of discouragement coming from the so called experts, it was no wonder that he had little desire to work for a miracle. He was the victim of a system that promotes external dependence and bypasses our internal power. This high tech system can be applauded for helping us live *longer* but there is only one system, our inner system, that can help us live *better*.

Supportive to a fault

In its wanting to help the needy and the oppressed, our society has in many cases become supportive to a fault. Its various systems support those who *can't* do for themselves, but it is also guilty of supporting those who *won't* do for themselves. Any system that suppresses, minimizes or ignores our natural creative power for change is no longer supportive. Many have argued that welfare has degenerated to supporting those who won't do for themselves. Contrary to common knowledge, the same is true of our Health Care System. The "we will take care of your every health need," (a definite misnomer), sums up the trademarks of health insurance companies, hospitals and pharmaceutical corporations. We have been led to believe that aside from good nutrition and regular exercise, (which 80% of people resist), bottom line, the responsibility for our health belongs to someone else.

Society cannot be totally blamed for our learned dependence. There is a tendency, some call it 'human nature,' to fight, defer or deny responsibility. The concept of responsibility has erroneously become synonymous with burden, blame and fault, of which God knows, we have more than our share. What is ironic, is that burden, blame and fault, the primary feelings associated with responsibility, are in reality the opposites of responsibility. Then again we shouldn't be too surprised at incorrect definitions; health has become synonymous with illness. Responsibility too often brings up the fear that we might be blamed for something. "It's not my fault," is one of the most common defenses heard today. As long as being responsible carries with it the burden of having to be right and perfect, (opening us up to rejection if we are wrong), then we will gladly surrender it to anyone who will take it. And for a price, there are a whole slew of systems and companies who will gladly do just that.

So where did responsibility get so poisoned with paranoia? This negative association to a most positive principle can be traced back to our childhood. Remember as a child, (it happens even now as an adult), when Mom, Dad, a teacher or anyone who we held in authority shouted our name. Before we could blink an eye or consider a belief, the fear of fault rang in our heads. The response, mentally or verbally of "What, what did I do?" became the standard defense. Sometimes all it took was a look from someone who was an authority to us - chin down, eyes raised, lips pursed, hands on hips - to send a panic up our spine. As we have subconsciously picked up this behavior and use it on our children and spouses today, do we wonder where our children, who subconsciously imitate us pick up such defiant behavior? The point, of course, is that the fear of fault - what some people call the *fear of responsibility* - keeps our unlimited creative power working at the minimum daily requirement.

Blame - the antidote for responsibility

Blaming everything and everyone - the government, the educational system, health care reform, our bosses, our spouses, our parents - rather than take responsibility for our troubles or lack of success, has become the social norm; then again so has stress, emptiness and chronic pain; could there be a connection? Finding a person who isn't criticizing someone for something is a rare breed indeed.

Finding someone who takes responsibility for their life, that their life is their own creative expression, positive or negative, is even more rare.

Talk shows have become our most entertaining medium for spewing blame. Whether it is a show on racism or family disputes, the overall purpose is to find a place to dump our frustrations. The raging emotions confuse and diffuse the original issue, besides the fact that these yelling matches make for great amusement. When blame and anger are the overriding attitude, with both sides fighting to be right rather than responsible, everyone goes home with their original negativity. Trying to make someone else responsible for our angry or negative feelings only serves to preserve the negativity in us. Only those who have experienced the power of taking creative responsibility for how they feel and want to feel, would know how true this really is. Choosing between pain or peace, even in a horrible situation, is what Dr. Victor Frankl called the *last of the human freedoms*.

Dr. Frankl, the famous Viennese psychiatrist, in his book, "Man's Search for Meaning,"[3] proved the greatness of our gift of choice in the seemingly 'no choice' circumstances of World War II. Dr. Frankl, a Jewish psychiatrist in the 1930's found himself thrown into a Concentration camp. He saw, as did everyone involved, the most intolerable situations known to man. For many, suicide or death, was the only freedom possible. Caught in the terror and despair, Dr. Frankl believed that suicide was his only way to peace. For some reason though, he got an intuitive sense that even in these unbearable circumstances, where every person was physically imprisoned and tortured, with little hope of rescue, freedom and even happiness could be found. Externally, those in the camps were stuck. But internally, in their minds, hearts and spirits, they *could* be free. Their bodies were subject to suffering, but in truth, no one could touch their inner most self.

---

[3]   Mans Search for Meaning, Victor Frankl, 1946 Simon & Schuster Inc.

Despite all the pain, Dr. Frankl found a way to inwardly rise above the circumstances that crushed the spirits of so many. By doing this, he and several others discovered a part of themselves that surpassed the pain and suffering. It was in this place that happy memories could be retrieved, new visions created, and a loving presence felt. Dr. Frankl recalled how he would remember the good times in his life, his wife, family, holidays and things that gave him joy. He often envisioned himself up at a podium telling thousands what life was like in the concentration camps and the spiritual joy that was possible even in impossible situations. Not only did these visions give Dr. Frankl a reason to go on, but years later he did find himself lecturing to the thousands that he had dreamed about.

Dr. Frankl also realized there had to be some meaning for this whole horrible situation, a reason that he had to be there. As a psychiatrist, all the books and test cases in the world couldn't reveal to him what he had learned from this experience. Dr. Frankl concluded that the gift of choice, regardless of any outer condition, was the *last of the human freedoms.* Even when circumstances are going far worse than we had hoped, we can find meaning or purpose in our life. In the case of the concentration camps, it was up to each person individually (their responsibility) to find a place where supreme support could be found and joy could be created. Only then would their suffering have meaning.

The reason that we speak so often of Dr. Frankl's story is that it shows to the highest degree, the magnificence of the human spirit in the most impossible of circumstances. If people like Dr. Frankl could create purpose, peace and even happiness in their minds, given an apparently hopeless situation, surely we could do this in our life. Pain or circumstances are often beyond our control. Suffering, however, is determined by our *perception* of the pain. It is this perception (how we choose to feel), that is always within our control. Once we realize it is our responsibility to create the thoughts, feelings and visions that we want, only then is the secret to true freedom and lasting happiness found.

Dr. Frankl called choice, the *last* of the human freedoms because he knew through personal experience that a person could be imprisoned physically, but nothing could imprison us mentally and spiritually. This freedom of choice is far more powerful than the physical world. Those who rose above the intolerable circumstances described in Dr. Frankl's book should be admired for their heroic courage. But that was not the full purpose of Dr. Frankl's writings. He wanted to make a lifesaving and life supporting statement about the power and freedom granted to *every* human being. In essence he said that we don't have to be in a tragic situation to summon our inner strength. It can and should be used in every waking hour of life. We submit that the best time to work on health, for the greatest benefits is when we are feeling well. Dr. Frankl's findings agreed with those of Jesus, Moses and Einstein, who have revealed that our human heritage is to live an abundant, joyous life. Our own United States of America Declaration of Independence defines freedom as the right to the *pursuit of happiness*. Making intolerable situations more livable is one benefit of the power of choice. Let us not forget that turning the normal, tolerable situations into wonderful ones is also our privilege. Thanks to these great thinkers, we see that in using our freedom of choice, we can create greater degrees of happiness, peace and purpose, even in the *best* of circumstances. Although it has gotten lost in the self created pressures of today, our birthright is to be happy and fulfilled. There is a catch, however; it is each person's individual *responsibility* to get there.

Responsibility is not about fault, pressure or what we *should* do. Responsibility in the truest sense is about freedom, power and what we *can* do. The word responsibility means our *ability to respond*, or in other words our *power to choose*. It is this original meaning, our power to choose, regardless of the situation that makes us human and gives us creative control over our life. Animals do not have responsibility because they do not have the power to choose. They cannot reflect on a situation or create a new thought about it. Neither can human babies. Both are instinctually guided and cannot improve their situations to any great degree. In fact all they can really do is adapt to situations as they are. Animals never get beyond this stage; a human baby does. They reach a point by the age of two, three or four, where they can creatively think; where they can to some degree make life better for themselves. They are then in the beginning stages of responsibility or the power to choose. This quality of responsibility is a gift, a birthright granted only to the human family. It was not given to us as a burden, but as an opportunity to choose *both* our inner feelings and our outer life. The power to choose prevents one of the most frustrating and painful conditions known to human beings; feeling *stuck*.

Nothing kills off the inner and outer life force more, and therefore the breakdown of the body, than believing that we cannot move, that we are overwhelmed by circumstances. This *feeling stuck* is the only real form of suffering. On the other hand, nothing invigorates the life force more than feeling *free*, that regardless of the circumstances we can find or create a sense of purpose and joy. Only using our attribute of responsibility, our power of choice, can we experience the most longed for state of being; inner and outer freedom.

What Dr. Frankl called the *last* of the human freedoms, we call the *first*. First and foremost, we are responsible for how we think and feel, not only is this a freedom, it is a fact. As long as we have normal functioning of our faculties, we are always free to choose our state of mind. Most people, whether they take advantage of this freedom or not would at least agree that this is true. No matter how we may believe that he, she, they or it made us annoyed, scared or exhilarated, in the end the choice was ours.

What we perceive as the *cause* of our stress, frustration, pain or joy, is really the *source* of it. That is why two people can watch the same movie, eat the same food, have the same mother and experience completely different feelings about all of them. These feelings can also change from one day to the next. One day a certain situation, like being cut off on the highway barely registers a thought while the next day we have fantasies of torturing the person. If any of these things, people or situations were the *cause* of our attitude, as we have been led to believe, then they would affect everyone in the same way every time. But they don't, so it is obvious that a choice made, consciously or not, has the final say.

The people and situations in our life don't *produce* our feelings, they *reflect* them. Either these feelings are choices we are making at the moment or past belief systems that automatically come up when a certain stimulus is presented. These beliefs remain that way until we take the responsibility to change them. Meanwhile, life, in its purpose of helping us heal our unresolved pain and grow into wholeness, continues to stimulate old 'ill' feelings that need to be changed. Recognizing our 'ill' feelings, (that lead to 'ill' health), and creating those that are healthy and life supporting, (that lead to a *well being*) is our number one responsibility. It is also the one we neglect the most.

The responsibility to choose the state of mind desired does not mean to sugarcoat a situation, deny our feelings or suppress our pain, it means just the opposite. The first step in taking responsibility for our state of mind is to know what that state is, how we feel at a given moment. Taking responsibility for our feelings means we have to *feel* them. The problem is that denying or deferring our feelings has become the social norm. Either we say and even believe that we are *fine* when we are not, or we turn our hostility, guilt or fear on someone or something else. Either way, we try to silence the feelings in our mind while our body screams them loud and clear.

In today's society, criticism has become the national pastime. We can always find someone to agree with us when we blame our family, boss, economy or disadvantaged childhood for our less than desirable circumstances. Empty positive affirmations are not the answer, either. "I am filled with joy," "Love is the answer," or "God will prevail," when we are seething with anger, filled with guilt or scared to death, only serves to intensify the emotional war inside. It isn't always possible to find happiness in times of turmoil or uncertainty; we are responsible however, to find *ease*.

Ease. . . another name for health

The word *ease* means total freedom. In the dictionary it is defined as 'freedom from *pain* or *discomfort*; freedom from *labor* or *difficulty*; freedom from *care*; freedom from *restraint* or *formality*.' put in other words, if we are at *ease*, we are free from hurt or displeasure; free from struggle or stress, free from worry; free from restriction or standards. If we could experience a day without hurt, stress, worry or living up to standards, we would no doubt search for that feeling the rest of our lives. No wonder we are so fascinated with young children, or yearn to be back in our own childhood. Assuming that we had a normal childhood, those were the days of true freedom and ease. Rarely did we carry resentment, hurt or worry in our hearts. We had few standards. This doesn't mean that our early childhood was always happy or problem free. The reason that children are generally bright, fulfilled and happy is that they are in touch with how they feel, (they have not yet learned to suppress pain or put on a good face for others). They instinctively choose to find purpose and joy even during times of turmoil. They find little or no value in blaming someone or something else for their feelings. They are, for the most part at ease, free from hurt, displeasure, struggle, worry and standards. They are also for the most part, free from chronic health problems. Could there be a connection?

Unfortunately this natural state of ease eventually fades. Anywhere between the ages of three and seven, we as a child learned about the normal trials of life. We learned to feel and store hurt, grief, stress, and guilt. We learned to struggle against life and our feelings. We learned there were standards to which we still feel compelled to attain. In other words, we learned to be 'responsible adults'. (Not exactly Dr. Frankl's empowering definition of responsibility.) But in the process of storing unresolved pain, fighting life and our feelings, trying to be something for the approval of others, we lost our natural state of *ease*. We became *dis-eased.*

Dis-ease. . . why such dis-trust?

As with many other words like disorganization, disapproval, discontentment, the *dis* before a word just means *without.* The word disease, originally spelled as 'dis-ease,' just means without ease, far from the catastrophic definition that the word brings to mind in this society. In other words, when we have a problem in our body - from a tight neck to a spastic colon - we have a 'dis-ease,' a *lack of ease.* It means that in some part of our body we have a hurt, struggle, stress or discomfort, a lack of the natural healing freedom; mysterious or scary, this certainly isn't. But the thousands of fear inspiring, and humanly indifferent labels have turned a workable term - dis-ease - into disease, the synonym for panic!

We redefined the word dis-ease, a grossly misunderstood word. It is not the devastating term that society has 'labeled' it to be. Dis-ease means a *lack* of *ease* somewhere in the body. This definition will ease the fear and severity normally associated with problems; that in itself is a major step up. But it is only a step to the real burning questions. How does the dis-ease in the body happen in the first place and how is it prevented and eliminated? Does returning the word dis-ease to its original meaning help the healing process or is it just a great bit of knowledge to help us win at Trivial Pursuit? If we really look at the words ease and dis-ease, their definitions clearly explain the 'whole' nature of health and illness, physically, mentally and spiritually. Physically, they describe either a *freedom* from struggle, stress, restraint and pain in the body or a *lack* of this freedom; in other words, *filled* with struggle, stress, restraint and pain. We really need to dwell upon what physical *ease* - freedom from stress, struggle and pain - really feels like in order to create it. (We need not dwell on what physical dis-ease feels like; we know that condition all too well.)

Getting back to the 'whole' nature of health and illness, the mental and the spiritual part of our nature, answers the original question; how does dis-ease in the body happen and how is it prevented and eliminated? The answer is simple; if there is a lack of ease in the *body*, there must be a lack of ease in the *mind* or *spirit*. If there is a hurt, struggle, stress, pain or discomfort, (a dis-ease) on the out-side, and if we are in tune with ourselves, we will find a corre-sponding hurt, struggle, pain or discomfort on the inside of us; in other words we are dis-eased in some way with ourselves or our life. There is a fight or a resistance going on within. We are no longer feeling free or at ease within. Our body, being a physical output of the mind and spirit cannot be at *ease*, in other words, can-not be healthy if there is any disturbance within. The physical is not separate, except in our current medical approach, from the mental and spiritual. Hippocrates said that we must treat the whole per-son, body, mind and soul. Instead of the health industry being so obsessed with striving forward, it would be wise to research a bit backward.

Many modern day philosophers and holistic physicians state em-phatically that the mind and body are just different degrees of the same thing. Many have said that our immune system 'listens' to our thoughts and reacts accordingly; in essence, there is a 'mind' in ev-ery cell of the body. To be more accurate, we should call the mind/ body connection, the mind/body *oneness*. A *connection* leaves room for a possible gap or breach, but a *one*ness prevents excuses and exceptions. When we allow for even a few situations in which the physical is separate from the mental or spiritual, "oh, this illness has nothing to do with my feelings," the gap grows larger. Before long we will find more and more exceptions to this rule and eventu-ally the majority of our ills and problems will be back into the category of accidents, luck or the will of God. Once again we are asked to accept responsibility without exception; *if* we want to create health.

It takes a truly responsible person to avoid the trap of wanting their ill to be 'real'. People are often relieved when traditional medical practices confirm their ill as something that mysteriously happened *to* them instead of something that was created *through* them. These people feel relieved because they are relieved of all responsibility for the condition. They are also relieved of all power to change it. We can try to make exceptions, but there really aren't any to make. According to current scientific proof, at least 80% of dis-ease in the body, (headaches, muscle pain, neck tightness, stomach upset, back pain, heart palpitations, allergies and any other lack of physical ease), is a reflection of the dis-ease in the mind or spirit. Today, no one in their right mind would disagree with the mind/body connection, consciously anyway. Subconsciously though, we fight this principle hoping that *our* ache, pain or ill is the exception to this rule. The price of pride over principle, wanting to be absolved of all responsibility for the condition is losing creative control over our own health. When we begin to see that in most cases all it takes to get back to physical ease is to create mental and spiritual ease, why would we throw away that kind of power? If by some remote chance, our condition *is* the exception, that it had nothing whatsoever to do with our thoughts, beliefs, feelings or expectations either before or after the condition occurred, (we would have had to be *unconscious* for that to happen), then we are still ahead of the game. By looking to heal the mental and spiritual dis-ease and return to an inner ease, another term for 'inner peace', at the very least, we would be far happier, at the very most, we would be far healthier. We can't lose unless we still want the responsibility for our body to be taken totally out of our hands. But *why*?

A message of mind/body oneness

A powerful example of this mind/body oneness came from listening to a message on an answering machine. Thirteen years ago, Doreen was a hurt looking to happen. Hoping to get a message on her answering machine from a particular someone, when it came, it was not the one that she hoped for. She expected this person to express how anxious he was to see her, but due to a misunderstanding, he expressed his desire to cool off the relationship instead! Within seconds, even before she had heard the whole message, her body finished the story. Without thinking, she became achy all over, began running a fever with the glands in her neck swelled to twice their size. In less than a minute she was 'sick'. All from an answering machine! Becoming so dis-eased with what she had heard, the body responded immediately. This incident was by no means a coincidence and although emotionally dis-easing, the message behind the head wrenching message was worth the pain. It was a real hands on experience showing how we direct the power of the mind through our emotions to heal or harm the body. To Doreen, this mind/body concept was no longer a possible theory, it was a fact. The dis-ease in her body lasted a week, just about how long it took her to let go of the anger and hurt. When peace was made with the whole scenario, a sense of ease returned and the flu symptoms began to disappear. Years later, she did get even with the guy on the answering machine, she married him!

Everyone has had similar mind/body 'messages', whether we are consciously aware of it happening at the time it is happening is another story. We have all become dis-eased outwardly, whether we call it a flu, a stomachache or blocked coronary arteries from being dis-eased inwardly. There may have been other contributing factors and the time between the emotional upset and the physical manifestation might have been days, weeks or years, but to deny a connection between the inside and the outside is to deny one of our greatest sources of growth. While we have been led to believe that the body mysteriously breaks down and that illness is something to be fought and feared, this theory goes against the higher purpose of our being. The wisest philosophers past and present, have told us that we are meant to live in joy, physically, mentally and spiritually. The body becomes one of our best guideposts along the way. When it is in *ease*, we are on the right track, with the purpose and potential of our being. When the body is dis-eased, a change, usually mental or spiritual needs to be made, a change that heals not only the *body*, but the whole *being*. While we may think the *body* is in pain, it is nothing compared to the anguish and suffering we go through when the mind and spirit are in pain. The body, being so much the object of our obsession, diverts our attention away from our real purpose in life (to heal the mind and the inner self), in other words, to become one with our Divinity. Instead of this grand purpose, however, the body has become the be all and end all of our existence. Because of a gross misunderstanding of health and the part it plays in our human growth, instead of a barometer (an indicator of pressure and changes), the body is seen as an isolated effect. That misinterpretation has almost cost us the whole purpose and potential of our existence. Fortunately, Emerson, Einstein and many of our modern minds refuse to let us lose sight of this truth. The body when viewed correctly, is our road to freedom. This freedom is our right; getting on the road to this freedom is our responsibility.

If there is a greater purpose to physical pain and discomfort than just random suffering, and an opportunity to find true freedom and joy in our life, is it not worth the effort? Simplifying the health crisis down to *ease* and *dis-ease* would allow us far more creative control over our health and the whole nature of our being. For a little more responsibility, we gain a 'whole' lot more life and life more abundantly. This new idea of *ease*, although the most natural approach to health, is far from normal. In this society, we have become accustomed to believing that we can secure health through someone or something on the outside and that the health care industry can keep us well. With that as our belief, working from within will seem like a waste of time. We have been led to believe that the better health insurance (promoting more affordable doctors, drugs and treatments), the better our health. If this were true, our health problem would have been solved decades and billions of dollars ago. Sick and tired of the false promises, a growing consciousness today knows that health is not a product that can be 'insured' from the outside, but rather a natural outcome of the ease or dis-ease; the flow or resistance inside.

What 'being' responsible really means

As the truth about health and the role we play unravels, our real responsibility becomes clear. We may have thought that proper nutrition, adequate exercise and having good insurance pretty well sums up our responsibility for health; actually these are only the beginning. Our true responsibility is finding a way to *respond to life* with more ease. If we are *dis-eased* with ourselves or life, the healthiest of lifestyles will be powerless against the inner turmoil. Doing all the right things on the outside would be fine if we were a car or some other physical machine. But somewhere our Health Care System has to get it into their head that we are more than a body. We can 'do till we're blue' but it will never be enough. We are human *beings,* not human *doings.* Our responsibility, if we want to be healthy, is a 'whole' lot greater than we have been told. There is the *external* aspect (our doing), like eating right, exercising and taking time for recreation. This is usually where the 'health plan' ends. More important is the *internal* aspect of our responsibility; one that has been grossly overlooked. The internal aspect (how we *feel* and what we are *thinking)* either opens up or shuts off the healing power. It is the only aspect that creates the ease or dis-ease within. This book is dedicated to that neglected internal aspect of our health. Jesus, one of the greatest healers of all time said to those who were ill, "Your sins are forgiven you, now go out and sin no more." He knew the power of a person's *feelings* on the inside; he also knew that these feelings, causing a frustration of the Divine flow, were the root of all problems, health being no exception.

More than anything, Jesus realized that in order for a person to "sin no more", they had to be educated on the laws of their being - the physical, mental and spiritual laws - so that the same dis-easing mistakes would not be repeated. Two thousand years later, the story has not changed all that much. We still need to realize that our negative feelings are frustrating the Divine healing power. And we still need to take responsibility for learning the laws of our being so that we can "sin no more." Do we still believe that we can bypass the truth of the ages with the mechanisms of modern technology?

The two aspects of our responsibility, the *external* and the *internal* (what we do on the outside and how we think and feel on the inside) are the most natural and most powerful sources of healing. Unlike any pill or treatment which has a shelf life of usually less than three years, these two aspects, (what we do and how we feel), have stood the test of time. The day is coming when instead of first prescribing a drug, doctors will say to their patients, "Take these two aspects and call me in the morning!"

To feel is to heal

Let's take a closer look at our internal responsibility; especially how we *feel*. Through our years of research we have read many books and heard hundreds of tapes proving the healing qualities of love, forgiveness and compassion. We also know how anger, fear, hatred and other negative feelings can make us sick. We agree but there is a vital step that comes before changing from negative to positive. Trying to rip out the anger from our hearts and stuff in the love, especially before we have resolved the dis-easing feelings is both stressful and ultimately, impossible. Repressing or manipulating our feelings as though they were an alien part of us is unnatural and unlawful (as far as the laws of our being are concerned). Before we can *change* how we feel, we have to *feel* how we feel. We are taught in this society that only the 'good' feelings, like love, happiness and patience are allowed. The rest, the socially unacceptable ones, like anger, fear and hurt should be sat on, controlled or ignored. Try sitting on, controlling or ignoring a volcano; do we really think all that energy will just go away? Hardly. It is only a matter of time before the pressure cooker of unresolved, unfelt feelings explode, with our body being he innocent bystander. Seeing the whole picture, (our Health Care System has omitted a few frames), it is no longer a surprise when the 'sudden, out of the blue', headache, sinus attack, stomach pain, pulled muscle or rash pops up. Does this mean that we should now blame ourselves for the dis-ease in the body now that we know it was the dis-ease in our mind that caused it? Only if we want *more* pain. It cannot be said enough that blame leads to guilt and guilt, as Jesus proclaimed, is the root of all of our problems. Blame leads to guilt but *responsibility*, responding to our feelings with ease and a positive solution, leads to Divine power. Taking true responsibility for our health means being responsible for our thoughts and feelings. Responding to our thoughts and feelings by *feeling* them is the only way to become at *ease* with them. And only when we are at *ease* can the healing power flow through in all its glory.

So, can anyone have ease or inner peace or is it reserved for the lucky or those people who have something that the rest of us don't? Actually, ease filled people do not have *more* of something than those who are frequently dis-eased. They do not possess more intelligence, earn more money or practice more religion. Actually it is the *less* that they have that makes all the difference; *less resistance*.

Resist not evil. . .

After all the struggle, striving, and worry in health deemed as *preventative*, do we have to ease up on all these feelings? Aren't we supposed to fight with all our might the enemy of dis-ease? No. If we continue in this vein, we will win the battle (temporarily) but lose the war. Resistance on any level, even for the most justified of reasons, dams up the healing power and there are no exceptions to

that rule. Jesus was one of the first to say it although his lingo was
and still is quite misunderstood. He used the term, "resist not evil,"
meaning "don't fight the negative." Everyone has at least heard that
principle. Yet the core of our life revolves around resistance, pushing till we drop, trying like mad to reach all our goals and still we
never feeling that we quite did enough. Of course there is a global
resistance that no one can deny. People fighting each other has become the social norm, but that is a whole other issue. The resistance to which we are referring is more subtle and far more
dangerous. That is, people fighting *themselves,* although not really
spoken about, has become the social norm.

It is not the negative feelings that dis-ease the body, it is the *resistance* - fighting, suppressing, forcing - of these feelings. It cannot be stressed enough that resisting and fighting our feelings is the
main cause of stress. And stress, another name for dis-ease, according to even medical authorities, accounts for over 80% of all
ills. Resist not evil means *fight not pain.* Ignore not, as well; find a
way to make peace or come to ease, perhaps not with the circumstances, but at least with our *feelings* about them. If we cannot
come to *ease* we cannot come to health. To find our way to *ease*
on the inside, (free from pain, discomfort, difficulty, labor, care, restraint or formality), is our primary responsibility in health. But
what do we do with all these pent up feelings? How do we relieve
the pressure and worry that begin and end our day? Where do we
put the guilt that never seems to end? How do we resolve the anger and hostility that has been with us since childhood? What do
we do when we feel so taken advantage of and hurt? Society has
certainly come up with some suggestions.

The 'easy' way out

"Relax." "Lighten up." "Just let it go." "Don't worry, be happy."
"Enjoy every moment." How often have we been told these clichés
by well meaning friends and family? How many times have we

given out these suggestions ourselves? But in the end, do they really help? Telling someone who is consumed with anxiety, riddled with guilt, annoyed to the max or fighting back tears, to just 'chill out,' is like a husband telling his wife in the last stages of labor to 'hold off' while he changes film in the camera. It just ain't going to happen.

In our controlled, put on a good face society, where what is happening on the inside is considered far less important than how we appear on the outside, a part of us is being shut off. Feelings, like worry, guilt, hurt, anger and self criticism, are for the most part considered socially unacceptable. We try to deny, defend or fight these feelings, do anything but *feel* them. This holding back of the inner part of us causes such an uncomfortable, unsettled state that except for winning the lottery, happiness and freedom are virtually lost forever. And even less realized, holding back or resisting of love can be just as dis-easing. Feelings are feelings; all are essentially Divine; the acceptable and unacceptable categories came from the human kingdom. Categorizing, denying or repressing any of our feelings leads to resistance, (there can't be one without the other), and resistance leads to dis-ease. Uniting, accepting and flowing with all of our feelings (pain and joy alike), makes us *whole again*. Coming into a oneness *within*, (the step before trying to find a oneness with others), uniting with all of our feeling, is what 'wholistic' or holistic healing is all about. It is not about eating organic foods or using herbs to heal our ills. Whole health is about becoming one with the whole of our being. It is through this wholeness, and only through this, that we can ever hope to heal the holes *in* us and the dis-ease outside of us.

If we refuse to listen to our feelings, our body does the talking. Thank God for that fail-safe; the illness is trying to lead us to wellness. Physical dis-ease, whether a cold or colitis, does not mean that the body is turning *against* us. The body is always working *for* us, urging us to get in touch with how we feel. Why? Because it is in this connection, becoming whole with ourselves that joy, peace

and self fulfillment - *true health* - are found. As we become more
at *ease* with our feelings, this connection and our wholeness become greater.

Does this state of ease mean that we roll over and play dead?
Hardly. It is not about ignoring the pain that has been stimulated by
other people or situation; we may have legitimate grievances and
things may need to change. The goal, for our health's sake is to
find a way to *release* versus *resist* the dis-ease we feel on the inside. From personal experience, we have found that once we become at ease with *ourselves*, the hurt, fear or anger that we thought
had come from the person or situation automatically lessens, if not
disappear completely. Maybe the dis-ease was with ourselves all
along? This is the most difficult concept to realize, it is also the
most healing.

What would life be like if we were more at ease? Can we imagine a
day of inner calmness, feeling free as well as completely secure, not
even thinking about the opinions of others, yet having the highest
opinion of ourselves. Are we willing to take responsibility for creating this case or would we still rather blame the economy, government, our finances, germs and all the irritating people in our life?
Blaming the world is still the social norm, then again, so is suffering. Before we blame the outside for our inside pain, and dis-ease
our body or our life even further, let us remember Dr. Frankl. He
and so many others found a sense of ease in circumstances where
death seemed the best alternative. If he and others were able to
"resist not evil" in the most horrendous of circumstances, we can do
it in the least of them.

Just listen to me

"Will you just listen to me." As a young person, how many times
had we felt that no one was listening, that our feelings, needs and
grievances were not being validated? How many times do we *still*
feel this way? Rarely is the grievance what we think it is. For

example, furious with our mate for coming home late, (so we think), we can't seem to shake the anger even after they apologize. Why not? After much self reflection we may find that it wasn't the lateness that angered us but what it represented; that our mate didn't really care about our feelings (so we believe). When our feelings are validated, the anger and the hurt that overpowers our good judgment are gone. Just by hearing "I understand how you feel," the cycle is complete. Feelings need to be listened to and they will be satisfied with nothing short of that. Will we still get bothered if our mate comes home late? Perhaps. Will it still enrage us? Only if we are not yet listening and validating our own feelings; the outer trouble is only reflecting the inner one. Is it someone else's responsibility to validate our feelings? Not really. It can help, but until we get to the core of the dis-ease, "*us* not listening to *us*," another person can stand on their head and spit nickels and we will still feel ignored. Our need to be listened to from others only echoes our need to be listened to by ourselves, however, now we can take it as a good warning sign to stop and take inner notice. When that cry is heeded, when we embrace our feelings (good and bad), with love and understanding, *ease* flows so *easily*.

People need to talk, or rather be listened to. And it doesn't take much for the dam of feelings to break. More often than not, old, unresolved hurts, fears, guilt and resentments, usually stemming from early childhood, are at the root of our pain today. As adults we try to rationalize them, but the child within continues to hold the pain. Feeling the pain as though we were once again a child helps greatly to heal the pain we have been harboring as adults.

The hunger to be listened to, a hunger that so few have been able to satisfy, is a signal from within to be healed from within. Listening with love and compassion to our own feelings, as would a doctor or a friend, fills the emptiness and satisfies the hunger. We were given the *ability to respond* to all our needs, problems and desires; we were also given the *responsibility*.

'Going with. . . not 'giving up'

The objective with ease is nonresistance, to flow with or surrender to everything we feel. Flow means to *go with,* not to pretend something isn't happening. Surrender means to *give up to a higher power,* not just to *give up.* *Going with* and *giving up* to a higher power, although odd behavior for controlling type personalities, starts us on a whole new path of healing. This flowing and surrendering are often the only healing we need.

Reclaiming our responsibility for how we feel on the inside, is going to take some getting used to. At first it may seem like we are giving in or allowing others to get away with hurting us. We may even feel that no one else is taking responsibility making us feel like we are doing all the work. The key to remember is the rewards for taking responsibility is inner freedom and radiant health. Once we get a taste for life without pain or strain, inside and out, swallowing our pride goes down much easier.

Who would have thought that trying to defer responsibility for our turmoil was in the end responsible for our headache, tight neck, chronic heartburn, high blood pressure or agonizing allergies? When someone innocently says that holding on to anger (irritation, annoyance or sensitivity as well), is a 'sick' way to live, we can now take that literally!

The R-I-D-E to Ease

Who would have thought that there would be so much 'B.S.' to clear up before the real healing could begin? And we are not quite finished with the 'B.S.' yet. However, it doesn't hurt to slip in a few healing truths along the way, especially since this book is not just an "it is" but also a "how to", if it is important enough to *do,* we offer a "how to."

Whether the dis-ease is physical as in the form of an ache, pain or illness, or emotional as in the form of anger, worry or self condemnation, the healing is the same. Healing on any level is attained only in the state of *ease*. We offer a four step process, using the acronym **R-I-D-E** as an 'easy' way to return to ease and a highly effective way to maximize our healing. Each of the letters in **R - I - D - E** - denote one of the four steps. '**R**' for Relax. ' **I** ' for Identify. '**D**' for Drift. '**E**' for Elevate.

(1) Relax. At the first sign of physical pain, tension or emotional stress, we are to get into a position, physically and mentally where we can *relax*. Closing our eyes and getting into a comfortable position may help, but if we cannot do this at the time, a few deep breaths will work. Imagine the muscles in the body, head to toe, releasing all tension. Breathe through the nose slow and deep. Exhale the tension out through the mouth. The key is to get as *relaxed* as possible given the present circumstances. Stay with this step until a feeling of ease returns, even a small degree.

(2) Identify. The next step is to *identify* the pain or stress. If it is physical, isolate with the mind the area of the body that hurts. Isolate it until it becomes an area of interest; for instance, "Isn't this feeling unusual." Do this until the area of interest becomes more of a *sensation and less* of a *suffering*. Without fear or anger about it, *feel* the pain. Most people think it is better to fight, deny or fear the pain. But pain in the body is either a pleading for healing or a path to it, and that vital message cannot be silenced. Think of the pain as a positive message and be open to hearing it. If the pain is *emotional*, an anxiety within, isolate it in the same way. What is the feeling, hurt, pressure, guilt, anger, disappointment? Get as close to the real feeling as possible. Many times the real feeling is far different than we originally thought. Anger may be covering up hurt. Pressure may be covering up fear. Guilt may be covering up self condemnation. The closer that we get to the real feeling, the easier will be the release; 'listening' to ourselves is the key. Continue this step until the isolated discomfort has eased a bit.

(3) Drift. The next step is to *drift* with the pain or problem. Every dis-ease, mental or physical has a cycle. If we interrupt that cycle as we can with drugs, denial or fear, it cannot be healed. *Drifting* with the pain, going with it, flowing through it without resistance lets the pain or discomfort run its course and release of its own accord, (it has been proven especially with childbirth, that pain intensifies when we fight it or try to pull away from it; it also lessens when we let go of it.) Drifting with a sensation, allowing it to move as it will is the path toward true 'letting go.' It will feel like the pain or distress is actually leaving the mind or body; we will begin to feel distanced from it. The inner or outer dis-ease must take us to the healing instead of the other way around. Drift until there is more ease than dis-ease.

At this point in the four step process, if we have done the steps honestly and thoroughly, the dis-ease should have partially or totally subsided. These first three steps are designed to *release* the dis-ease, but this last step is to *heal* it. True healing means that there is a shift in the being, a shift toward a permanent change, the ultimate goal. Who wants to heal the same problem day after day?

(4) Elevate. To *elevate* means to get *above* the pain or discomfort, to create a mental image of what we want. If we could only 'see' how much we had been creating a mental image of the pain (what we *don't* want), we would be amazed. (If the picture doesn't change, neither can the pain.) The most vital point in this step is to visualize the body or mind without the problem and then to picture how life would be when this happens. Get excited about the new healing; true healing is the most exhilarating of all feelings.

Although to elevate is the final step in healing, it is interdependent on the first three. Trying to elevate ourselves above the pain before we have really felt it will only serve to intensify it. We need to first free the pressure that surrounds the pain before healing can occur. Rushing this process, skimming through the steps, or avoiding them totally, only prolongs the pain. Can we see now why pain or stress goes on in many cases for a lifetime? We have never fully completed the healing cycle! The whole four step process, *Relaxing, Identifying, Drifting, Elevating*, once practiced takes only a few minutes and within time becomes automatic, a new belief. The goal is to eventually become so adept at riding out the pain that ease and radiant health become our natural state.

A R-I-D-E a day keeps the pain away

Practice, it really does make perfect. The R-I-D-E of healing, becoming more at ease inside and out just requires practice, everyday, several times a day, if possible. Do it now as the message is still hot. And if we think, "But I haven't got any pain or stress right now," think again. We may have become so numb to the pain and distanced to the stress that we *think* that it isn't there. Let us not delude ourselves. The pain and the stress that we *think* isn't there is killing us. Like a slow gas leak, we may not see it, smell it or feel it, but the damage is being done just the same. As we use this R-I-D-E process, we will know how numb we have become, not just to the pain but also to the pleasure. The R-I-D-E will open up an ease, energy and exuberance of which the numbness has robbed us. 'Feeling' again is the best feeling possible. We will never know how much we have been suffering with pain, (even if only slightly), until we feel the long lost exhilaration of living without it.

We can argue till the cows come home, no matter how justified or how much we may feel the world owes us something, the responsibility for our feelings, no less our health is always ours. This does not mean it is up to us to make things happen, we are not the healing power and we are not God. Our job is just to get into a receptive state where both can flow. Einstein said it best. After years of research to discover the solution to both universal and individual problems he said, "You can't expect to solve a problem with the same thoughts you had when the problem was created." He seemed to understand the benefit of the responsibility, the *power to choose*, to choose the new thoughts that create the new condition. That is our responsibility, our most important responsibility and one that only *we* can do. Whatever the manifestation, from guilt to gout, we choose the thoughts that either open the healing or stop it. We can refuse to accept that responsibility and continue blaming the things and people in our life, but the effects will stand. There will be no change until we change the thoughts that we had when the problem was created. And there is no exception to that rule.

Shift Happens. . .

If we are satisfied with our lot in life, our health most specifically, then we will not be so inclined to rethink this new level of responsibility. But if we have realized the miraculous healing qualities of responding to life at a higher level, and we are 'sick and tired of being sick and tired', we are ready. Responsibility, our 'ability to respond', is not something that we *must* do, it is something we are *meant* to do. The power to choose any feeling and ultimately any condition that we desire is our human birthright. Nothing will ever be as precious as this gift. The gift is ours when we accept the responsibility for it.

'B.S.' # 2: The Health Care System *can* and *should* be responsible for our health should now seem rather ludicrous. Can they still help? Of course, so can welfare. But if we rely on either system to 'do it for us', welfare or health care, neglecting our own unlimited power; then mediocrity or *not too sick* is the best we can hope for. Is the majority of our society ready to accept this truth? No. But there are those of us who are starting to shift. Those of us who take the responsibility now, even if the rest of society thinks we are nuts, are the only ones who will feel a health shift like never before. As soon as we accept our responsibility in healing, *shift happens.*

'B.S.' # 3:
Good Health means not being sick

"Raise your hand if you think you are in good health?" This direction is given during a group exercise. 80 - 90% of the audience raise their hand to affirm that they are definitely in good health. "OK," raise your other hand if you try to do all the 'right things' for health, like eating well, exercising, taking vitamins, cutting down or eliminating caffeine, nicotine and the sun, as well as keeping abreast of the latest health warnings." About 80 - 90% of the audience raise their other hand. "We've run out of hands, so this time, raise your leg if even though you do most if not all of the right healthy stuff, you still get headaches, backaches, allergies, high blood pressure, problems with your stomach, sinuses or any other part of your body. " This time instead of a show of hands, there is a 90% or better show of feet. Watching all the faces wondering what will come next, the audience is asked to raise their other leg if they believe that today's Health Care System will spend millions more of our tax dollars before they find a cure for these chronic aches, pains or the more serious ills, if they ever do. At least 90% of the audience raise their other leg. Wondering about the point of this 'exercise in stability,' we end the suspense by asking the audience to look around the room at the rather unusual spectacle. To all those with hands and feet in the air the question is posed, "Given its past track record, if we wait for the Health Care System to discover the 'magic pill' that will cure our aches, pains and ills, as far as current and future states of health are concerned, do we really have a *leg to stand on*?

Today's idea of good health just isn't 'good enough'

This group exercise always gets a good laugh, but the point to be made is quite serious; asking a person if they are in 'good health' is always quite enlightening for us. We have learned to abstain from asking this question at parties and family gatherings; those in our workshops seem far more open to the question. "Yeah, I'm in good health," almost everyone would say, rather matter of fact. "So, you have no complaints about your health, no health problems to speak of," we would ask. "No, not really," most would answer. And here is where the responses get real interesting. Usually before we could probe any further, the person with whom we are talking will add something like, "I'm in pretty good health. Oh sure I get the normal headaches and colds. I've had strep throat a few times, the flu again this year, but then so has almost everyone else around me. Oh yeah, my sciatica bothers me every now and then, my doctor says I have to watch my cholesterol, I've been tired a bit, but isn't everyone? Hey, I'm not complaining. There are people much worse off than I am. I'm healthy relatively speaking. Nothing serious, thank God."

Except for varying symptoms and labels (some had allergies, others got migraines) the majority of people with whom we discuss the 'good health' idea answer with the same general response. The majority of people start by affirming their 'good health.' When asked about any physical complaints, they rattle off their aches, pains and doctor appointed labels, almost as if they are a normal part of 'good health.' In the hearts and minds of so many today, minor ailments, like paying taxes, have become an annoying but inevitable part of life. As if to justify these chronic aches, pains and ills, many people will exclaim how 'things could be a lot worse.' Compared with the major health problems afflicting so many, our society has accepted a macabre sense of gratitude for the minor complaints.

If it closes us off to our birthright for truly living to feel grateful because we are not 'dying' is really sick. We have been led to believe that headaches, backaches, allergies, colds, tight muscles and the constant fear of getting sick are acceptable as long as they are 'nothing serious.' This book was written because we believe that striving for anything less than ease, energy and exuberance in our health is very serious.

Annual health check

Think about each question for a minute before answering. They may require that we get in touch with conditions in our body for which we have unconsciously desensitized ourselves. Remember, we can only heal from where we are, not where we think we should be; full awareness without criticism is the attitude we need to develop.

1) On an average, how many <u>days per week</u> do you have aches, pains, stiffness or muscle tightness, even slightly? _____

2) Multiply the above answer by 52 weeks = _____ days/year.

3) Add to the above answer the <u>number of days</u> within the last year that you were 'not feeling well'; you had a cold for a week, or the flu for four or five days, a 24 hour virus, a sinus attack for a few days, a two week bout of allergy suffering, a hospital stay or any other illness you get only occasionally.

$$\underline{\hspace{2cm}} + \underline{\hspace{2cm}} = \underline{\hspace{3cm}}$$
$$\quad\text{\#2}\qquad\quad\text{\#3}$$

4) Add to the above answer the number of times that you had to visit a doctor or health care facility (other than for a check up or maintenance), due to health problems. _____

5) *Subtract* from the above answer the number of days, if any, that you felt a definite flow of ease, energy and exuberance in your body that far exceeded the normal days of aches, pains, tightness or ills. $\underline{\hspace{2cm}} - \underline{\hspace{2cm}} = \underline{\hspace{3cm}}$
$$\qquad\qquad\quad\text{\# 4}\qquad\quad\text{\# 5}$$

The point of this most revealing exercise is to see in black and white how many of the 365 days of our year are lost to dis-ease, pain, discomfort or remedying them. Shocking to the senses, the numbers usually range from 120 - 180 days. This means that 30 - 50% of our year is drained by pain. What is most shocking is that these are the averages for people who are in 'good health' relatively speaking, God help those with poor health! We can continue to justify these numbers by saying that for the most part they do not reflect anything 'serious'. But nothing serious, just like good health, is a relative term. According to our natural potential for radiant health, living 120 - 180 days a year with aches, pains and ills, although considered 'good health,' is just not good enough!

What is 'good' anyway

Once again it has to be remembered that the seemingly radical ideas in this book are for a very select group of people. They are for those who want the best in every area of life, health being no exception, and are willing to accept full responsibility (along with the help of others) to get there.

The idea of 'good' is a relative term. For some, a 'good marriage,' means freedom, love and sincerely caring about one another, for others it means that arguments are kept to a minimum and basically we tolerate each other. A 'good financial situation' to some means that money is always flowing to afford all that we need without the least bit of stress. Others think it means just about making ends meet every month. By not realizing their divine right to inner peace and fulfillment, many feel that they still have a fairly 'good sense of self' even with daily guilt, self-criticisms and self-doubt. And compared with those who are clinically depressed, this standard is *good*. But why are we looking *down* if we want to raise ourselves *up*?

It may take a while to raise our standards beyond what the world calls 'normal' to our birthright called 'natural,' but by seeing how low these standards have become, we have a great start. Just

imagining about a better life and redefining good as far more than
not bad, sets the positive forces of nature in motion. Although it
has taken a beating over the last century, health is no exception to
this rule.

Half empty or half full

Remember the two schools of thought that we have been brought
up on? We can look at life in two ways, *half empty* or *half full*.
The first, half empty, obviously signifies the *limited* way of thinking; it shows that a person looks at life negatively, always waiting
for the other shoe to drop. The person who sees the world through
half empty eyes starts defeated, with a 'life gets worse before it gets
better' attitude. Knowing a little about the power of thoughts we
see this kind of an attitude is not a *prediction* of the future as a pessimist might contend, but rather a *projection*. Through a person's
state of mind the forces of nature are set toward the 'I never get a
break,' attitude. And to no great surprise, they never do.

Of course those of us who consider ourselves positive attitude people endeavor to convert the pessimist into the eternal optimist. We
try to change the half empty, hopeless attitude into the socially preferred, half full, hopeful one. There is one fatal flaw with this philosophy, one so subtle that it has been consistently overlooked. It
is true that the attitude of half empty is limited. But to say that the
attitude of half full is therefore *unlimited*, misses one vital point.
Although seemingly opposites, both are based on the idea of *half*.

Unlimited versus 'less' limited

This 'half' point will make more sense as we translate it into today's
trendier terms. Half empty and half full have been updated to the
terms *dysfunctional* and *functional*. We hear so much about dysfunctional relationships and dysfunctional families, that although
only a decade or so old, it has become quite the '90's term. It has
become so normal that a great majority of people have affirmed that

they either are in or have come from a dysfunctional situation. Similar to the half empty/half full, the goal is to turn dysfunctional situations into those that are *functional*. But also similar to the half empty/half full concept, turning dysfunctional into functional uses only *half* of our potential. Functional, like half full is not *un*limited, it is just *less* limited.

Whether we are talking about health or wealth, there is a whole un-tapped side of our potential. It is not *half* anything nor is it merely functional. The idea is based on the idea of *fullness*. Using the trendy terms, many modern philosophers call the other side of our potential *fully functional*. Instead of just being less limited or not as bad, fully functional allows for unlimited possibilities. The point of *un*limited versus less limited, fully functional versus more func-tional, is not based on greed or an incessant need for perfection. The purpose of fully functional is to open us up for possibilities that we in our often too limited thinking could not imagine. Fully func-tional means that a power greater than we is assisting and guiding us toward an abundant life. Our responsibility is to get into a posi-tion to be receptive to this power. Beginning to think in terms of *fully functional* is the first step.

Many of our ideas about what is normal fall under the heading of good (relatively speaking), or what we are now calling functional. All areas of life have suffered from these rather limited norms but none as painfully as health. These norms keep us physically *func-tional*, feeling okay, no 'real' complaints, dealing with the pain. And if functional health is enough, (we either do not desire more, cannot imagine more, or will not accept the responsibility for more), wait-ing for the Health Care System to *give us more* will frustrate us all the more. When there is a raise in consciousness or as philosophers term, a 'paradigm shift' from functional to fully functional, there will be a corresponding raise in health. There are no exceptions to this rule.

We think therefore we are

Too many people unknowingly take a creative approach toward life that is functional at best and dysfunctional at worst. They see a situation in a certain way, hear a suggestion from someone else or diagnose a certain symptom in their body and *at that point* decide their thoughts.

These thoughts, being creative energy, then recreate the same situations, suggestions and physical symptoms as were thought about in the first place. It is not the circumstances of life that create our thoughts, ("I would feel wealthy if I had more money and healthy if I had more ease") but it is our thoughts that create the circumstances in our life. We would have more money if we thought wealth and more health if we thought ease. Isn't it ironic that most people spend more time planning the activities for their day than the thoughts for their life?

This 'thought to circumstance to thought to circumstance' cycle would actually enrich our life if we took the *fully functional* approach, that is, if we held a Divinely guided hopeful, joyous, faith filled attitude balanced with thoughts of the kind of health and life we would like to have. But until there is a course in our schools called "Fully Functional Living 101" and until there are parents who have attained to some degree of *fully functional* living themselves so they are capable of teaching their children, it is unlikely that we will wake up each morning with a fully functional song in our heart.

Due to the 'half full' standards in society today, there is scarcely a person who thinks above the *functional* or *dysfunctional* approach. Here is where the trouble begins. If a person approaches life dysfunctionally, with a generally negative attitude, believing that life gets worse before it gets better (if it even does), feeling almost powerless to change any present or future condition, gives up often, then they and their life can't help but function at a dysfunctional level. Fortunately, the majority of people do not fall into this category. Most of us have risen above the standard of poverty and have created instead a standard of mediocrity; we are *functional*.

Functional is as functional does

It can't be said that a person who is *functional*, who takes a functional approach toward life has a negative attitude like the dysfunctional person, (at least not outwardly). On the contrary, the *functional* person (probably most of us), struggles to make things work come hell or high water, burns out before giving up, leaves no stone unturned, yet feels stress and pressure at every turn, wants to make it 'big' although they think rather small, believes that there is always a solution to all their problems, even though there is always a problem to be solved. Those of us who strive to remain functional no matter what is thrown our way almost always do.

Clearly taking the functional approach to life is unquestionably better that the *dysfunctional* one. But comparing mediocrity to poverty leads to another question. Why must we be limited at all? We don't. But in order for our life to be unlimited, our approach and our thinking have to be raised. Both the *functional* and *dysfunctional* approach 'react' to life, although the former reacts with a better attitude. Nevertheless, reaching such conditions leads us to base our thoughts on how we see our life; the level of thoughts and of consciousness remain about the same, and year after year, so do the conditions of our life. It is only when we create our thoughts and our paradigm of life independent of the current circumstance that our consciousness and our future circumstances will be raised. A *fully functional* life is open to anyone who will approach it that way.

The three approaches to life

These three approaches, dysfunctional, functional and fully functional are the ways with which we consciously or unconsciously create our life; we reap today that which we had sown yesterday.

As Jesus said, "by their fruits ye shall know them." Using the more modern terminology we say, "by the effects in their life you will know their approach." We could also say, "by their state of health you will know their thoughts." Each statement is saying the same thing; we can tell a person's state of mind or approach to life (dysfunctional, functional, fully functional) by what is happening in their body and life. Isn't it a relief to learn that all we need to do is live by a higher approach and the rest takes care of itself? "Let go and let God" is a miraculous principle but let's at least give God a great foundation from which to work.

Modern day philosophers freely use the idea of *fully functional* to describe a person's potential for financial success and even self actualization. But when it comes to health, the term *fully functional* is fully ignored. And if this term is not happening in our mind, it cannot happen in our body. In our teaching, therefore, we use the three approaches to life in everything; success, relationships, spiritual growth and of course, health. A principle is a principle regardless of the desired outcome. For the purpose of this book, the focus will be on how these three approaches either *expand* or *expend* our health. There is no 'right' approach to life; all three are within our free choice. If *functional* results are satisfactory, (one day good, one day bad, much stress with occasional spurts of success, minor but frequent health problems), then a functional approach is enough. If, however, we desire *fully functional* (most days are great, much success with only occasional spurts of stress, radiant health is the norm), then it would be foolish to expect these results with anything less than a fully functional approach. We are always free to choose the creations in our life, but we are absolutely beholden to the results of our choice. There are no exceptions to this rule. Thank God for that.

If we look at health on a scale from 0 to 100 as we would at any standard in life, something strange is revealed. Instead of working from 0 to 100, from *no health problems* to a grand state of *radiant health*, the aim for health in our society misses this mark by a hundred miles. The goal is to get to '0' health or no major health problems. Living without the threat of getting seriously ill sounds good, but is it good enough? For some, being able to meet their financial obligations every month, living without the threat of getting into serious debt, is enough. For others, having debt is not enough, these people want financial abundance. In the same sense for some, living without serious ills is not enough. Many people want to finally get beyond '0 health', (not being sick), and begin working toward 100% health, (being really well).

The Line of Health

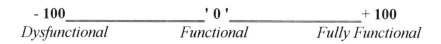

- 100	' 0 '	+ 100
Dysfunctional	*Functional*	*Fully Functional*

This line is only an illustration of where each approach or category falls, but it gives us an idea of the limiting boundaries placed on health, as well as the higher potentials that are rarely considered. To be *functional* with regard to our health, the previously acceptable high is mediocre at best. As we desire more, we will realize that *fully functional* health is only a few degrees away.

THE THREE CATEGORIES AND APPROACHES TO HEALTH

DYSFUNCTIONAL ("Sub Normal")	FUNCTIONAL ("Normal")	FULLY FUNCTIONAL ("Natural")
Reactive	**Curative/Preventative**	**Creative**
1) dis-ease, pain and/or fatigue is frequent	dis-ease, pain and/or fatigue is on and off	ease, energy and exuberance is frequent
2) pain or dis-ease *dysfunctions* life, disabling 'normal' activities	pain or dis-ease *drains* life, but still able to 'function'	energy and ease *invigorate* life; life is fuller more complete
3) daily fear & anger	daily stress & struggle	daily joy & fulfillment
4) focused on *fighting*	focused on *fixing* problems	focused on creating health
5) attitude is one of hopelessness	attitude is one of hoping	attitude is one of hopefulness
6) surrender to health problems	surrenders to health care system	surrenders to healing power within

Let's review the categories going straight across the board. The subheadings, *"SubNormal," "Normal," "Natural,"* cause us to think that what is considered 'normal' is not always the best state in which to be. Particularly with health, the 'norm' is well below the level to which our being is naturally predisposed. And if something is 'natural' to our being, and the laws of nature are followed, this grand state is the easiest, most effortless to attain.

The subheadings *reactive, curative/preventative and creative* describe the general concept with which we knowingly or unknow- ingly view health. Reactive - waiting until a problem arises and react emotionally either tries to get rid of it or attempts to deny it - it is the *dysfunctional* approach. Dysfunctional relationships, those in which abuse or addiction become the central theme are handled in the same way, (waiting until the problem arises and then trying to get rid of it or deny it). Higher in the scale, curative/preventative, means preventing a health problem *before* it happens or attempt to cure it once it does. Both preventing and curing use physical meth- ods to treat the physical body. Much of the focus of our present day Health Care System is to prevent or cure serious ills. While this is certainly better than waiting until the problem occurs, the *functional* way, doing everything we can 'not to get sick' still keeps our health far too limited. This may not be the dysfunctional ap- proach but neither is it the *fully functional* one. More effective than either curing or preventing illness is *creating health.* The *fully functional* creative approach uses more than physical methods to get to more than 'no illness.' Creating radiant health is the main purpose. This approach finally allows us to create what we *want* for our health, a condition that is the secret to our health but one of society's *best kept* secrets.

The health chart is split between the effects and the cause; rows 1 - 3 are the health effects and rows 5 - 6 are the approaches taken that caused the effects. (Row 3 is actually the pivot point as it can be seen as both effect and cause).

Row (1) describes the physical state of health within each category. As might be expected, under the *dysfunctional* category, there is frequent dis-ease, pain or fatigue; a condition of constant suffering that just about defines daily life. Most of a person's thoughts and actions would be centered around their pain or ill. Obviously, no one would want to live in this category if they could help it, but to assume that *functional* health, even though considered normal is the best to hope for, assumes too little. On again off again dis-ease, pain and fatigue, even though far less frequent is not the way our being was intended to live. Living with *functional* problems may not consume *all* our thoughts and actions as does *dysfunctional*, but even a little is too much.

The *fully functional* category shifts the potential for health to a whole other level. Frequent ease, energy and exuberance characterizes *fully functional* health, a state far more natural and far more appealing than on again off again pain.

Row (2) shows how our state of physical health affects the whole quality of life. Obviously living with *frequent* pain or problems would definitely dysfunction life as a whole; having to adapt life around the health condition, (instead of the other way around, would severely limit normal daily activities.) The real limitation surprisingly occurs in the *functional* category. It has become so normal to believe that good health means we are able to 'function' in our daily life. What about the subtle but never-ending drain that on again off again dis-ease, pain or fatigue has on our life? This so called normal state is well below our natural state. Yes, even a little dis-ease will drain our life as a whole but the opposite is also true. *Fully functional* health, filled with energy, ease and exuberance automatically invigorates our life as a whole. In fact just as our state of mind influences our health, our state of health influences our quality of life. A body that surges with ease and energy would surely make for a more joy filled existence than one that aches, cramps and becomes exhausted half way through the day, no matter how slightly.

Row (3) displays the emotional demeanor of a person in each category. This is a pivot point because on one hand it shows the *cause* of the physical state of health while on the other it shows the effect. For example, in the *dysfunctional* category, constant fear and anger, will contribute greatly to chronic or serious physical dis-ease, pain and fatigue. Similarly this physical pain and suffering will, if not dealt with, reinforce the fear and anger; a vicious cycle that cannot be changed unless the person changes. No surprise there. The surprise once again occurs in the *functional* category. It has become so normal to go through the day with emotional stress and struggle and to believe these states are far better than the fear and anger that we have come to accept as a necessary part of survival. Yes, we survived but the so-called normal stress and struggle break the body down. Just like fear and anger, only just a bit slower. This aggravating but 'livable' state of health (a little pain here, a tight back there), leads to more stress and struggle. It is impossible to be peaceful and joy filled with a splitting headache. This state may be perfectly normal, but it is a far cry from perfectly natural.

Looking at the *fully functional* category, we see that there *is* another state in which to live. Daily joy and fulfillment, a choice just like stress and struggle, creates the physical state of ease, energy and exuberance. If it is no more difficult to choose joy and fulfillment than stress and struggle or even fear and anger, why don't we? We certainly couldn't prefer pain to peace, why then does the latter seem so many rungs above us? The answer is no different than for any common condition in our society; it is society's *conditioning*. Stress and struggle are such common topics of conversation, we can describe them in vivid detail while living in joy and self-fulfillment would require a refresher course before we could *talk* about them intelligently. Although far more natural to our being than stress and struggle, it would be difficult, maybe impossible to describe in detail a joyous, fulfilling life; a joyous and fulfilling day might even take some deep thought. And if we cannot think it, we cannot be it. This comparative illustration was designed to change all that.

The last three rows show the attitude and approach that create the corresponding quality of health. Row (4) shows that a person in the *dysfunctional category* generally fights or resists the physical body; they blame all the suffering in their life on their 'bad' body. A person in this category will contend that the pain and suffering will probably never end, so their only choice is to hate it or fight the body. This attitude is certainly understandable given the degree of suffering. But it is the continued resistance of the body that keeps it in pain and suffering. No matter how it may appear otherwise, it is *attitude to body* not the other way around. And even a *dysfunctional* body can be healed by a more *functional* to *fully functional* attitude.

The *functional* person although seemingly less dis-eased in their life, suffers in much the same way as the *dysfunctional* person, the only difference is that their suffering is more subtle. Instead of out-wardly *fighting* physical pain or dis-ease, this person concentrates on *fixing* it. The *functional* approach is to fix health problems as they crop up and they do over and over again. The focus of heal-ing, both in the cause and the effect area is on physical remedies for healing the physical problems. There is little or no unifying of the inner person with the outer body, nor is there much concern with the healing of the inner person. This of course sustains the state of on again off again pain, dis-ease and especially fatigue; there is al-ways a subtle resistance of even slight or unconscious physical dis-comfort. This state of minor but chronic dis-ease cannot change as long as our body is fixed in pieces. Healing of any *piece* of the body requires healing the being as a *whole*.

In order to attain *fully functional* health, the ease, energy and exu-berance that make our life soar, a 'whole' different approach is ne-eded. Constantly fighting and fixing the physical, with drugs, treatment, check ups (the 'normal' plan for health) will never induce this upward shift. That is why few people in our society can hon-estly say they have *fully functional* health. . . yet. Healing the *whole being*, physically, mentally and spiritually, is and always has been the easiest most natural plan for health and contrary to popular 'health' belief, the only real *cure*.

Row (5) illustrates the three ways in which hope is used. Hope is a powerful tool in healing of any kind whether it be for health, wealth or any other area of life; there is something magical about this energy. Hope in the truest sense, (this is another principle that needs some redefining), can heal the most devastating of situations and bring a degree of peace to anyone at any time. It is our hope, however, that the magical energy of hope is not reserved just for times of trial. True hope, another natural part of our being, brings about a sense of joy unmatched by any external thing. A truly hopeful attitude, as in the *fully functional* category, can move mountains. By the same token, a hope*less* attitude as in the *dysfunctional* category, can start an emotional and physical avalanche. We can live without many things in life and still survive, even excel. Hope is not one of them. Hope*less;* feeling completely overcome by inner and outer conditions with no visible or 'invisible' light at the end of the tunnel, sucks the life out of us. Few people would deny the sickness of hopelessness, but to believe that we as a society understand the full scope of hope is only wishful thinking. Obviously staying far away from hopelessness, regardless of the circumstances that seem to justify it, is a healthier way to live. The principle of hope, unlimited in its true capacity has been reduced to the idea of *hoping*, wishing that life would get better. Although it may appear to be of a positive attitude, 'hoping' or 'wishing,' is generally based on inner fear and even a subtle sense of hopelessness. That is why people of this mind set spend years 'hoping' things will change, only to be disillusioned by the fact that they rarely do. This is because too many of us confuse the inspiration of *hope* with the desperation of *hoping*.

True hopefulness, the natural state of our being, means that we are *full of hope*; there is an inner knowing, (although no external proof may have yet appeared), that life *will* get better. Hopefulness is an inner state of being in which we live and breathe, not just an emotion that we call up in times of trouble. You'll know the difference between being hopeful and merely hoping; the former will bring a sense of peace before and regardless of the outcome, while the latter will keep us anxious and worried until the situation is resolved. True hope or being *hopeful* is the goal. Being full of and filled with hope is more valuable and blissful than anything we can *hope for*. True hope is a Divine state of mind and doesn't just give us what we want, it is what we want. Hope is the opposite of worry and living the opposite of worry is easily the most peaceful way to live. True hope, knowing that the Divine energy within us has solved and healed any and all problems of life can also be applied directly to our health goals, regardless of where we want to be. And as can be expected, feeling hope*ful* leads to ease and energy, while hop*ing* keeps a sense of stress and the on again off again ills always bubbling at the surface.

A true sense of hopefulness is concomitant with the surrender that comes in the last row. Row (6) shows where we put our faith for health and healing. In the *dysfunctional* category, there is no faith. A person who follows this approach to life and health surrenders to the problems at hand, feeling completely overwhelmed by them, and thinks constantly of these problems. This of course keeps the pattern of frequent pain and dis-ease in a never ending cycle. Faith in and surrendering to something greater than ourselves is absolutely vital to our sense of peace as well as the success of our goals. But if that 'something greater' is limited to a man made system, we are not only kidding ourselves, we are cheating ourselves.

No, having no faith or surrendering our life to problems is no way to live; it will eventually fulfill its own prophecy. In this *functional* approach, we surrender our healing to our Health Care System. This system is well equipped to treat maladies of every kind. But for the person who wants to wake up and live every day with ease, energy and exuberance, the *system doesn't work*. This is not to say that outside systems cannot help; they can be a great support *in addition* to our own internal system. The final change, however, takes a source far greater than anything that can be artificially created on the outside. Surrendering to the healing power within vs. an external system make the difference between a *functional* and *fully functional* life.

We may never have seen health categorized or approached in quite the way that this chart has illustrated. Then again we may not have ever been told that *fully functional* is fully within our right and our power. Of course, with this right comes the responsibility of creating the conditions in rows 3 - 6 in which it can grow. In a nutshell, the *fully functional* person 'creates'; the *functional* person 'waits' and the *dysfunctional* person 'negates'. The *fully functional* person creates the feelings and conditions in which they wish to live. The *functional* person waits for conditions to change before changing the state of his mind. The *dysfunctional* person negates most of what is happening keeping a consistently negative state of mind. These three categories and approaches are to show us where we've been. To change where we are going, we need to change the approach. (This chart gives us great benchmarks, it should be studied carefully and often.) There are additional attributes of health to be considered, like proper nutrition and exercise, but there are numerous sources from which to learn about these physical laws. We recommend the *Rays of the Dawn* book[4] by Dr. Thurman Fleet.

Bringing a forgotten radiance back to health

"Give me health and a day and I will make the pomp of emperors ridiculous." That is a quote from Ralph Waldo Emerson who strived for and believed in nothing less than radiant health every day. His was a time well before 'modern medicine.' Yet or maybe because of that, he had an innate sense that health in its most magnificent expression was every person's rightful heritage. Emerson put no antecedent conditions on radiant health, nor did he seem to

---

[4]   **Concept-Therapy Institute, 25550 Boerne Stage Rd, San Antonio, TX 78255, 1800-531-5628**

fear its loss. Maybe 'conditional health' is part of the modern problem. We place too many conditions on health, "if I eat this. . . if I
don't do that. . . when the government changes this. . . when a cure
is found for that. . ." And even after all this work to do the right
things, the ultimate goal, is 'not getting sick.' There is a far more
radiant state of which to aspire to than less sickness; God knows it,
Emerson knew it and now we know it.

In his book, *Return of the Rishi*, Dr. Deepak Chopra explains that
we have to want radiant health at least as much, if not more than
anything else in life. Emerson made health - radiant health - the
very foundation of his life. Dr. Chopra in his commemoration of
Emerson's health ideals, remarks that because we are so mentally
caught up in pain, sickness and disillusionment, we dismiss Emerson as an optimist, a 'Pollyanna'. But Dr. Chopra sees, as do many
proponents of this kind of idealism, that Emerson tried to do more
than make people 'feel' good, he tried to open them up to their
birthright. "Motivated by his own healthiness, Emerson aimed for
exuberant vitality in everything."[5] As he 'aimed for' he also reaped.
In essence Emerson believed that radiant health, natural to the human family, heals all weakness in a person and allows for compassion, joy and inner peace of the most self and life enriching kind.

The picture of health

Was Emerson more *fortunate* than we are or was he just more *focused?* Instead of just talking about the 'As you sow, you reap'
principle or denying it altogether, Emerson lived it. He made radiant health the very foundation of his life. What state of health is
the foundation of our life built on? If we opened up the head of
Emerson, Jesus or any great healer, we would see a vibrant faith inspired, life enriching picture of health. If we opened up our own
head, would the same picture be found? If not, let us spend time
each day beginning now, creating the picture of what radiant health

5   **Return of the Rishi, Dr. Deepak Chopra, Houghton Mifflin CO, Boston**

means to us. We are in a great position to become the 'picture of health'. All we need to do is *picture this health.*

Radiant health or
ravaging health problems

Radiant health is certainly not the normal topic of conversation. On any given day we can listen to the news on TV warning us of a deadly new virus, scan billboards across the highways with 800 numbers cleverly created with the name of the dis-ease and we hear family, friends, and cashiers at the supermarket discussing their aches, pains and recent hospital stays. With these stimuli bombarding our senses, a most crucial question must be asked. Is this rather bleak and pain filled picture of health the *result* of the kind of health problems we see and hear everyday or the *cause* of them? Which came first, the sickness or the *sick image?* Could we not see a dramatic shift in health, particularly from *functional* to *fully functional* as we shift our perspective from the fear of ravaging health problems to the freedom of radiant health?

We can choose to wait until modern science proves this principle of 'mind over matter,' and then wait another twenty years for them to study the effects. But who has that kind of time? It might be wiser to shift our focus from health problems to healing power. And let us do it now while we are in fairly good health. It cannot be overemphasized that it is much easier to *grow* well than to *get* well.

So, this is good health?

As we have seen, health is a 'relative' term. (Ask any of your relatives, they would be glad to give their view.) If we relate our minor but annoying aches, pains, tight muscles and occasional ills to those people with serious problems or constant suffering, then we can safely say that we are in 'good health'. This concept of 'good health' (no real problem) has been accepted as the upper echelon, a state in

which one should feel lucky to be. On the other hand, if we relate
our minor dis-eases to people like Emerson whose health had a
definite radiance about it, we can safely say that our idea of 'good
health' is *not good enough*. As long as we adhere to the belief that
health means not being sick or not being *really* sick, we will accept
our relatively minor suffering as *not that bad*, creating nothing new
in our minds to reflect nothing new in our body. This will leave us
with a certain sense of melancholy because deny it as we may, pain
no matter how relatively minor, still hurts.

No matter how much proof comes out to support our birthright for
radiant health, it will take patience, perseverance and persistence to
relate to and create such a grand state. Even if we accept this radiant new view of health *consciously*, ("Yes, I believe that"), subconsciously where the 'B.S.' can be found, the old conditioning is
rock solid. It will take time to chip away at the rock until nothing
but a pebble of fear exists. And even if we are not currently worried about our health, thanks to the panic inspired approach of our
society, all it takes is one physically ill symptom to get our ball of
fear rolling. Healing our sick image needs to be done whether the
'B.S.' is rumbling or not. Still waters run deep.

As far as changing from *dysfunctional* to *functional* to *fully functional*, accepting success can be a bit uncomfortable at first. And in
this case, health is *not* the exception to the rule. A person who has
struggled financially for years, no matter how much they believe
that they want financial success, may find it extremely uncomfortable to accept it. The same is true for people who have lived for
years with turbulent relationships. All of a sudden being treated
with love and respect after years of feeling unlovable or being
abused, can feel strange and even stressful. The same can be true
for self esteem, weight loss, even spirituality. When unworthiness,
no matter how unfounded surrounds a person's inner most self, 'getting the best in life' will take some definite 'getting used to' (more
will be explained in Part III, "The transition".)

If we are not aware of this human belief in suffering and most of us are not, we will unconsciously sabotage the very goal that we so desperately desire. Although few have ever considered healing and unworthiness in the same context, health is no exception to this rule. Tightness, tiredness and tension, traits that are often found in the good health *functional* category, have become so normal, that subconsciously we cannot imagine living without them.

From our personal experience, *functional* pain was a constant in both our lives. Each of us suffered with a constant pain and stiffness in our neck. There were many reasons for this constant 'pain in the neck,' none of which were because of too much cholesterol, second hand smoke or the draft in the house. The reason the problem remained chronic was the mental picture. Although quite subconscious, when confronted we could not *imagine* life without this pain. As with any habit, after a while we just became numb to it and even more, we *expected* it to happen. It wasn't until we created a state in which the pain was far less that we realized how much we had been suffering. Recognizing (feeling) the outer pain, healing the inner pain and creating a mental picture of *no* pain filled our heads and necks (and of course of minds) with glorious ease. Give *us* health and a day and we can make the pomp of emperors' (or the need for material things), ridiculous.

If you can feel it you can heal it

In order to shift from our *functional* state of livable aches and pains to our *fully functional* potential of ease, energy and exuberance, we have to feel exactly where we are right now. This is a rather strange request since in our society pain is believed to be the enemy and to be avoided at all costs. This is definitely the normal approach to pain but not the natural one. Pain is not the precursor of doom as many people have been led to believe. Pain is a call for healing, a signal to quiet down and listen. In order to heal it we need to *feel* it. Read the rest of the paragraph and then do the simple exercise. Close your eyes and relax with a few deep breaths.

Notice without any emotions where if any dis-ease becomes notice-
able in your body like a tight neck, throbbing head, aching back,
upset stomach, etc. Feel the dis-ease wholeheartedly.

Unless they have been in serious pain, most people are surprised at
the subtle discomfort bubbling just beneath the surface. "I never
knew my shoulders were so tight," or "I can't believe my back aches
like that," are some of the remarks made during this exercise.
These people became consciously aware perhaps for the first time,
of the 'normal' dis-ease that constantly gnaws at our body and our
life. Can we continue living a fairly *functional* life with this discomfort? Unless it becomes more dysfunctioning, most of us do. So
too can we live a fairly *functional* life with frequent financial
struggles, vacillating self esteem and discordant, but tolerable relationships. As long as these areas do not become so bad as to render us *dysfunctional* we can live a relatively normal life. But is
normal *good enough*?

Radiant health. . . can you imagine?

"Can you imagine," has become such a common aphorism when
talking about something foreign to normal life that when analyzed it
reveals a subtle but powerful truth. The imagination, considered by
many rational adults as 'child's play,' is actually the predecessor of
physical results. "As you can conceive and believe you will
achieve," is one of the most powerful principles carried down
through the ages. This principle expresses the power of the imagination, certainly not just kid's stuff. If we want to live in the true
radiance of health, we must imagine it in all its glory.

Fully functional health has many different degrees. The basic
premise is that it *adds* to life rather than drains it. How *much* it
adds to life is up to us. The point to keep in mind is that logical,
gradual growth, rather than a frantic shot in the dark is far more effective. The degree, depth and feeling of our health goal is completely up to our imagination. For some, less pain or a release of

some of the tightness and tension is more than enough. Others, not suffering from any pain whatsoever, may be ready to experience a new surge of energy and vitality. The key is flow, not force. A consistent, steady evolution is the best way to insure radiant health for a lifetime. We have seen too many 'flash in the pans;' people who set out to reach radiance by the end of the week, only to fizzle out at the first hurdle on Monday morning.

The R-I-D-E to radiant health

At this point we may be saying 'radiant health sounds incredible, but who has the time?' Living in a world where struggle and hard work are seen as the keys to success, it is difficult to imagine something wonderful happening in our life freely and easily. Health, even radiant health is just such an effortless thing. The free flow of unlimited health and healing is one of those human gifts that takes no effort at all, adds immense happiness to our life, rewards us in ways yet to be imagined and once achieved will never forsake us. We may not have been taught this truth until now, but our being is destined toward radiant health. Believe it or not, we have to work very hard *not* to be healthy. Unfortunately this is just what we do. Getting ourselves to a state where the unlimited healing power has an open, unclogged channel in which to flow is a natural process and takes no effort.

The R-I-D-E exercise discussed in 'B.S.' # 2 will be beneficial when beginning to experience radiant, *fully functional* health. Read the rest of this paragraph before actually doing the exercise. We will be going through the four R-I-D-E steps.

(1) Relax mind and body for a moment; deep breathing, 4 - 5 times with eyes closed will help. (2) Identify the part of the body that hurts or aches. No effort is needed as the dis-ease will reveal itself. (3) Drift with the ache or pain allowing it to freely move where it wants to go. Drift until it eases up. (4) Elevate to a state of health that is logical but improved; a gradual but definite raise in ease.

Here is where the imagination kicks in. We must decide exactly how we would like our body to feel. It can be a release of the tightness and pain. . . a wonderful sense of ease where the ache or pain had been. . . ease all over the body. . . renewed vitality and pulsating energy flowing through the body. . . an enthusiasm and happiness in the body that adds a sense of joy to your whole being. Choose one of the above images, or create a whole new picture. As clearly as possible, (it will get clearer each time we do this), imagine this new state and *feel* it with the whole being. Take a minute to *fully* experience this elevated state of health. Imagine now how much better we will feel waking up in the morning, going through our day, doing the simplest of activities of living, but *really living*.

Radiant health. . . an 'out of body' experience

Describing the experience of greater and greater degrees of health to someone who at best believes that 'good health' is not being in major pain or with a serious ill is like trying to describe a gourmet meal to someone who lives on fast food and frozen pizza. It is impossible with any amount of beautiful words to describe the difference between 'good' health and 'radiant' health. It is more than a physical or verbal experience; the whole being, body, mind and inner self are affected. With science today trying to simulate sensations through high tech movies, biofeedback and interactive techniques, we tend to think that the heart of our needs and desires can be artificially met. We cannot speak for every sensation, but regarding an exalted state of health, 'virtual reality' just doesn't cut it. As Dr. Chopra writes in his book, *Return of the Rishi*, "health should be not simply strong but invincible. It should be so perfect that nothing better can be imagined and nothing worse can touch it." Now that's an advertisement for health!

Radiant health is our responsibility to humankind

While radiant health brings a sense of joy that makes getting up in the morning a renewing experience, the effect it has on all other areas of life is just as miraculous. No one would argue that illness and pain diminish the quality and performance in every area of life, but how many of us realize that the opposite is just as true. *Fully functional* health, where we feel like a million, has a radiant effect in every area of life. Not only does the surge of physical ease and energy cause us to work at a higher level as well as act more patiently and harmoniously, but there is a most positive effect on others around us. The positive, radiant energy exuded from this healthier state lifts the spiritual essence of everyone with whom we come in contact; even if no words are spoken.

"The universe is the property of every individual in it. It is his, if he will. He may divest himself of it; he may creep into a corner and abdicate his kingdom, as most men do, but he is entitled to the world by his constitution", says Emerson. Dr. Chopra commenting on Emerson's ideals says, "The constitution of man, his mind and body, tunes him to the universe and gives him title to it. If Emerson is right in this, we had better start looking more closely at what it takes to assume our rightful possession; it takes health. Only that. But *perfect health*, pure and invincible is the state we have lost. Regain it, and we regain the world."[6]

And to think that our health care system is working day and night to create a drug or treatment that will eliminate serious illness, to get us back to '0,' *functional* health. Whether or not there can ever be a drug or any other artificial method that will cure all the illness that currently plague us is another debate. For this discussion, however, considering the perfect health ideals enunciated by Emerson and Dr. Chopra, with the corresponding effects on life, *good health* as it relates to not being sick, is definitely *not good enough.*

---

[6]   **Return of the Rishi, Dr. Deepak Chopra, Houghton Mifflin CO, Boston**

If we are to ever attain that exalted state to which Emerson referred, claiming our birthright to the universe and lifting the mass
consciousness in the process, then perfect radiant health is not only
our privilege, it is our creative responsibility.

'B.S.' # 4:
Healing is from the body
and for the body

All of society's Belief Systems have contributed in their own special
way to our own personal level of health. If we are satisfied with
our current level of health and feel secure for the future, (no wor-
ries, anxiety or confusion about health and illness), then 'B.S.' # 4
will not be of much help. If however, we are *not* satisfied with our
current level of health, (we want less pain or more radiance), and/or
we are *not* secure with how our health will play out in the future,
hearing 'B.S.' # 4 will take the dis-ease out of our heads, if not our
body.

'B.S.' # 4: Healing is *from* **the body and** *for* **the body** is all the
'B.S.' about health rolled into one Belief System. We are led em-
phatically though subtly to believe that healing comes *from* the
body, (by doing something physical to the body), and is essentially
for the body; what else needs healing except for the body? This
well accepted, continuously practiced, though rarely evaluated approach is not only illogical, it kills the whole idea of wholistic
health. The terms, physical, mental and spiritual are not just to be
used for evolving our conversations; they are to be used for evolving our consciousness. It is wonderful that *body and soul* sound
bites advertise everything from a week long retreat to a brand of
yogurt. Society has become more comfortable with saying these
words but beyond that, most are way out of their comfort zone.
Regardless of its long odds and short term success, the physical approach to healing (healing the body *from* the body) and focusing on
only the physical needs for healing, (healing reserved only *for* the
body), remains standard procedure. It also remains the standard
'B.S.'

What's wrong with this picture?

Let's face it, our society is obsessed with being 'health conscious'. We are on 24 hour patrol against cholesterol and have sworn off everything from caffeine to nicotine. Exercising until we are blue in the face, we hope to outrun sickness and sagging. On guard for every warning sign from being unduly tired to overly wired, the stress and worry about staying well is killing us! While we may be 'doing all the right things', instead of radiating with health and energy, too often our body hurts more than it heals. Something is definitely wrong with this picture!

What _do_ we believe?

In our workshops, the reaction to this last 'B.S.' is generally one of shock and awe. On the surface, the participants agree wholeheartedly with taking a real wholistic approach to health. But health beliefs have a way of showing up at the most inopportune moments; when we are sick or scared. We believe in testing our beliefs in a more controlled environment; when we are well and secure. A workshop exercise called "How we get sick and how we get and stay well" is geared to get an answer not from what we've learned but from where we live.

The objective in this exercise is to write up to ten things that society teaches and we still tend to agree with (even slightly), that cause sickness and create health. In order for this exercise to help heal the 'B.S.', we tell people to write down only those things that they truly believe (even if recent new information is making them questions these things). It is suggested not to include those things that have just been learned, but rather those that have been accepted for years.

How we get sick   **How we get and stay well**

_____   _____
_____   _____
_____   _____
_____   _____

The answers. . . truth or 'B.S.'?

We have used this exercise for several years in our workshops. The answers rarely differ from audience to audience. Many would say this is a major coincidence; we say it is a major conditioning. The majority of us in society come from the same school of thought, the same 'medical' mindedness. Even those of us working on a more wholistic 'whole being cause and cure' approach may still be run by the 'B.S.' of the past. It is crucial that we pull out the 'B.S.' before we try to shove in the truth; we can't fool our inner nature.

The following are the generally given answers in order of potency to 'how we get sick'. See how they match up to yours.

How we get sick
1) Germs from the environment
2) Germs from other people
3) Viruses
4) Smoking
5) Bad genetics / family history
6) Eating high fat foods / too much caffeine
7) Lack of exercise
8) Pollution / toxic waste / pollen
9) Change in weather
10) Stress

The list looks fairly 'normal.' In fact, unless a person were from a totally different culture or had been studying wholistic healing for years, they would agree with this list without hesitation. It covers all the bases, germs, smoking, high fat foods, stress; the Surgeon General would be proud. Whether these answers are actual truths and whether knowing them so well has really kept us so well, is up for major debate. But before we analyze this sick side, let's look at the answers we have gotten over the years to 'how to get and stay well.'

How we get and stay well
1) Medicine
2) Quitting smoking
3) Watching for the warning signs / regular checkups
4) Good nutrition
5) Regular exercise
6) Rest and relaxation
7) Don't get stressed

This list is about as 'normal' as the first list, nothing out of the ordinary. The only surprise to us, no matter how often we do this exercise, the audience always knows many more ways to *get sick* than to *get well*. We actually stop the group when they get to ten ways to get sick. They could go on 'ad nauseam' because almost everyday a new health no-no is discovered. Unfortunately, the audience usually cannot think of more than six or seven answers on the wellness side. Could that be telling us something? Definitely. Once again our society is so fixated on *curing sickness* - fearing it, checking for it, talking about it, labeling it, and coming down with it - there is little room to think about *creating health*.

An even more crucial point is revealed in this exercise, one that is probably responsible for how we get sick and how we get only *functionally well* than all the other answers put together.

Except for the last answer in each list, all the traditionally held 'causes and cures' focus on the physical, what we *do* to get sick and what we *do* to get and stay well. Without realizing it, society has taken this one dimensional approach - *from* the body - and made it the 'whole' of our approach to health.

A Matter of Timing

We still flinch when our programs are thrown into the category of 'wellness.' It isn't that our purpose is anything else but ultimate well being; we have spent more than a decade studying the principles behind a truly *well being*. The problem comes in when we are viewed through *society's* conception of health and well being. When we began our health quest in the early '80's, the minute that we told people of our wellness business, a conglomerate of interpretations emerged. "You must be an exercise program," many would conclude. "Not exactly," we would reply, "our program develops the *inner* and *outer* being." "Of course," people would say, "you do nutrition too." "No, actually we teach *holistic* health," was our next attempt. Thinking on that statement for a few seconds, the response would be something like, "Oh, now I get it, you're into vitamins!" After two years going in circles trying to explain what we were about we finally called ourselves a 'fitness business' and left it at that. Properly categorizing our service, we discovered early on, was impossible. A category hadn't yet been created to house us!

How society categorized our health business depended on the consciousness of the particular time. In the early '80's, health or wellness was almost a totally physical process. This was the time of the fitness boom where exercise was considered the antidote for illness. A few years later, nutrition - low fat high fiber foods and vitamins - became the cure-all. Although these choices definitely elevated our lifestyle and were far better than our sedentary, junk food habits, it was far from a truly holistic approach to health. Unfortunately, many people at that time believed exercise and good nutrition were the 'whole' picture. We dare say even with the acceptance of the mind/body connection, the thinking today has not changed all that much.

In the late '80's and early '90's, another dimension was added to society's quest for health. Shifting from the mostly outer approach of the past, an inner aspect was added. Our 'health' service was now seen as more than exercise and nutrition. Because of the changing times we were thrust into the category of *stress management,* a definite step up. Now when we talked about our program as an advanced approach to wellness, holistic in nature, at least the *mind* came to mind. Unfortunately, that is where it stayed. Emotions and stress were intangible in nature and far less understood than the very measurable aspects of exercise and nutrition. The mind was accepted as a major factor in *theory,* but when push came to shove, germs, cholesterol and drugs always won out.

Today in the late '90's, the mind is big business. Scientists and medical professionals agree that our mental and emotional state are direct factors in health and illness. Leading health magazines speak highly of managing stress, living with forgiveness and loving ourselves as health enriching ideals. Our society has a long way to go with regard to the mind and emotions in *practical* use - most doctors will quickly prescribe *medication* but rarely suggest *meditation* - but we are turning inward. In a manner of speaking, we are also turning *upward.* The spiritual dimension, developing a deeper connection with God and our innermost self, is being reviewed as a viable path to health. Prayer, inner communion and cultivating a more spiritual aspect of life are no longer religious issues. They are logical, lawful principles of life, *especially* with health.

The acceptance of mind and spirit regarding health is encouraging. Are these intangibles as widely accepted as cholesterol testing? Hardly, but spiritual fears have relaxed a bit. The word meditation does not cause the stir it did in the early '80's. But being comfortable *talking* about this higher principle of healing is one thing; being comfortable *using* it is a whole other story. Contrary to the beliefs of many regarding religion, following perfectly all the religious rites gives us no more rights to God than the person of no religion. We get no bonus points for *bowing* our heads before God, only for *filling* our heads with God or the power within. It is a state of consciousness that entitles us to life changes, not a state of religiousness. God or this power does not change our thoughts

(that is our job), but does create *through* them. It is what we believe with the whole of our being (something that we seriously need
to analyze), that creates the lot (or the little), of our life.

The spiritual dimension of our being - what we believe about a
higher power, our relationship to it and our real purpose in this life
- are not just good ideals to ponder on the Sabbath, but great ideals
to base our life upon. What a paradox; this higher dimension gives
us the most creative power and at the same time too often gets the
least of our attention.

Today we can freely talk about how stress breaks down the body
faster than any germ, or that prayer can aid healing in ways that
medicine cannot. But actions speak louder than words. When push
comes to shove, society pushes us back to traditional *physical* healing methods. If a symptom appears in our body, inner meditation
takes a fast back-seat to outer medication. Even the preventative
approach runs back to tradition. We are pushed to take our yearly
'physical'. When was the last time, however, that we were pushed
to take our yearly 'spiritual'?

Society converses about the mind, philosophizes about the soul,
and *lives* by the body. Herein lies the core of our problems. It is
true that we are *doing* all the right things, but the essence of health
lies not in our physical doing but in our whole being.

Once again, thanks to today's magnificent obsession with the body
and the physical attempts at healing, we have come to the last (but
far from least), of society's 'B.S.' about health. 'B.S.' # 4: Healing is
from the body and *for* the body pretty well sums up our problems in
health and our pain in life. We have been led to believe that health
comes *from* the body (by doing something to it), and that health is
reserved *for* the body (the body is the only aspect of our being
needing to be healed.) While that statement may ring perfectly true
to the masses, it should be hitting a sour note with us. If however,

the 'B.S.' in 'B.S.' # 4 hasn't quite hit you, the rest of this section
will make sure that it does.

The 100% focus on less than 20% of our potential

Although society still puts 100% of their focus on the body, in
truth, the physical aspect of us is at most, only 1/3 of our whole being. Society also limits the goal for health to *not being sick.* Going
back to 'B.S.' # 3, we recall that *not being sick*, is only 1/2 of our
full health potential; the other half is *radiant* health. Let's math this
out; if we only focus on the *body* and only as it relates to *not being
sick*, we have reduced our full 100% potential for radiant health to
1/2 (not being sick), of 1/3 (the body); 1/2 of 1/3 is 1/6 out of
100%. When we put all of our healing efforts on the *body*,
(nutrition, abstinence from nicotine, exercise, physical check ups,
drugs) and then only to prevent and cure *sickness*, (the success of
which with our traditional approach to health is quite limited) then
the best we can expect to attain is 1/6 or roughly 16.5% of our full
health potential. Our society spends billions of dollars on health
care for 16.5% of our health potential? We can get better odds at
the slot machines!

This current one dimensional approach of physical health would be
more than adequate if we were a *one dimensional being.* Were we
just a physical machine, a body, then physical things like good
nutrition, regular exercise, normal maintenance check ups and drugs
to fight off problems would keep us in perfect shape. But we are
far from a physical machine. At the least, we are three dimensional,
a physical, mental and spiritual being. A one dimensional approach,
even if done perfectly, just scratches the surface of our three dimensional needs and our three dimensional possibilities.

Studying the mind/body oneness has become a respected science,
and few level minded people today would refute its power in
theory, at least. We may not fully understand it or realize the

absolute 'cell to cell' effect that our thoughts have on our body (the science of psychoneuroimmunology can explain it best), but believe it or not, the inside of us is molding the outside of us at every moment.

Although the mind over matter principle is being studied at famous institutions by brilliant scholars, you don't need a Ph.D. to prove its merits. Examples of how our thoughts literally and immediately translate into our body can be seen by anyone and everyone. TV sitcoms have used this connection to get laughs for years. If anyone is a *Honeymooner's* buff, they will remember the episode in which Ralph and Norton wanted to prove their manhood by drinking an entire bottle of wine. Afraid that they would get sick, Alice and Trixie their wives, poured out the wine and replaced it with grape juice. Still containing the aroma of the wine, within minutes Ralph and Norton were plastered, barely able to walk and each went to work hungover the next day. Upon watching their husbands pass out, Alice and Trixie commented, "it just goes to show you what the power of suggestion can do." That was pretty bold for the 1950's.

Another example of the power of suggestion, another term for the mind/body oneness, occurred several years ago at a baseball stadium. After drinking a can of soda from a machine in the stadium, a spectator became violently ill and had to be rushed to the hospital. Trying to avoid further catastrophes, the management made an announcement over the loudspeaker that the soda was contaminated, possibly toxic. The announcement further described the symptoms that could be expected; vomiting, terrible stomach pains, possible fainting. Within minutes, scores of people began experiencing these same symptoms, some needing immediate medical attention. The powerful effect of suggestion, especially with panic winning out over logic instantly affected an entire stadium of soda drinkers. Even with such an instantaneous connection between the management's announcement and the spectator's physical sickness, no one even thought that the power of suggestion might be the real culprit.

But the story was not over yet. Within less than an hour, the soda in the machine was tested, as were many other foods sold in the stadium; no toxins were found. The test results were negative but the following phenomena was proof positive of the mind/body oneness. As soon as the announcement was made that the soda and foods were toxin free, the previously ill spectators became symptom free; nausea, vomiting and dizziness disappeared as quickly as they had come. Whether or not those with the appearing and disappearing symptoms ever realized the real point to this story isn't known. But someone had; it was printed in a magazine under the title "What the mind can do. . ."

Like the stadium example, the health reports that we hear every single day need not be in the least true (in fact, they are very often proven years later to be 'B.S.'), yet their effect on society is powerful.

The Panic Principle

Can we remember the last time we felt really spooked, let's say walking alone at night or hearing a strange noise in your house? In response to such a fear, a rarely observed phenomena occurs over our entire body. Believing on some level that we could be in real danger, that some evil perpetrator was about to attack, every muscle, joint, system and cell of our body instantly prepares to run or fight back; scientists call this the *fight or flight principle*. Our heart pounds intensely, every muscle in our body stiffens, our senses become keener just from a wave of emotion; essentially every part of the body completely changes. Even normal processes of the body like digestion and elimination are diminished to prepare for the run or attack. Most amazingly, when we have been assured that no one is lurking around and that we are safe, all these symptoms of 'dis-ease' (they certainly sound like some of the most heeded warning signs), subside.

Most of us dismiss the miraculous transformation in our body during the *thought* of attack as an isolated event reserved for these fearful situations. Few would stop mid panic and think "This is amazing, within a split second of my mental fear, my physical body went into attack mode. I wonder if the same phenomena occurs with other thoughts?" No, most people wouldn't see the principle for the panic. The principle of mind/body oneness, though even more subtle, is well proved when the fear is only two dimensional. The body cannot distinguish between one fear over another. Being afraid to give a speech can have the same effect as being afraid of being mugged. Remember a time we had to give a speech or even stand up and say our name to a group of people? There were no monsters or enemies around, yet if speaking in front of a group is a 'fate worse than death', our body will go through a rollercoaster of convulsions. Just thinking about giving the speech days before, can stiffen our body and increase our heartbeat every time we think about it. Just imagine what happens to the health of the body when fear, worry, stress or frequent irritation, the so-called normal struggles of life, become the mainstay of the mind.

Occasionally, we rise above the fear, (an occasion that should happen much more often), and connect with a power that knows no fear. Speaking of public speaking, Doreen remembers one that was as tragic as it was enlightening. Panic pretty well described Doreen's feeling of giving a speech in the late '80's. This particular one she not only had to give but write as well. The speech was called the "Real Self," but it was the 'Hark, I hear a cannon' syndrome revisited. Doreen tried for weeks to *come up* with a clever, entertaining speech on the "Real Self." It never occurred to her that she had to actually *connect* with the Real Self to write about it. Struggling, sweating, up until the last day, nothing but 'B.S.' came out on paper. She felt this had to be the worst thing that could happen to her. She was wrong. About 4:00 p.m., Doreen got a call that her grandmother whom she had seen the day before had died. It was devastating to say the least and more than put her fear of speaking into perspective. The fear along with much of her need to prove herself was at least for the time being, gone. Emotionally spent, she went to bed about 1:00 a.m. assuming she would sleep well past her 8:00 a.m. speech. She had told the appropriate people that she probably would not attend, so the fear and pressure were gone. Without the fear and without setting the alarm, she woke at 6:00 a.m. with a burst of energy. She then sat down and wrote nonstop, no changes, for 30 minutes. (In the last 3 weeks, she hadn't written a sentence.) When she gave her talk, it was given with as much flow and security as when she wrote it. The success of her talk was secondary to the lesson she learned. Nothing short of an inner power could have transformed her outer being so greatly. Nothing short of this inner power ever transforms or changes anyone's outer being.

Getting the juices going

To illustrate the mind/body principle quickly and definitely, we do another workshop exercise called the 'Lemon Test'. One person comes to the front of the room and sucks a lemon while the audience watches and winces. We ask the non-suckers in the audience to describe what they felt. Not surprisingly, even though they had not tasted the lemon, almost everyone in the audience describes an instantaneous salivation in their mouths. This, like the panic in the dark situation, rarely makes much of an impression on them. "So what if we salivate just by watching someone else suck a lemon? What does that prove?" It proves just about the whole nature of health and illness. Just the mental image of something, from a fruit to the flu, will cause a reaction in our physical body or life. As human, spiritual beings we are entitled and responsible to create the mental image that we want in our physical being, like radiant healing, strong teeth, glowing skin. We are also entitled to block out - become immune - to that which we *don't* want in our beings. Yes, we can immunize ourselves. The Lemon Test is then repeated, only this time we ask the audience to mentally *block out* the effects of the lemon. From thoughts of "no, I don't want this experience," to "I will not allow the lemon to affect me," anyone able to hold this immunity to lemonitis was completely unaffected by the lemon. Our point is to prove that pictures or broadcasts of this 'itis' and that illness can be coming from every 'health' expert that we encounter, yet we can hold fast to health. As long as we practice regularly creating the image of health, staying firm and secure in our right to be well all the time, we can block out the 'lemons' of sick suggestions that try to make us salivate to their 'B.S.' If our mind does not have the picture, our body cannot have the effect.

Our responsibility is of course to take time out to create the radiant, energetic body of ease that we *want* and spend time recognizing, blocking and healing our fears of illness. No doctor, drug or insurance company can do this for us; then again with the unlimited power in our own minds, who would want to put the healing in *anyone* else's hands?

Really getting the juices going

Everyone can relate to watching a sexy movie, reading an erotic book or thinking of a hot looking person of our persuasion and feeling quite 'in tune' with the experience. Even though we are not engaging in the act physically, the effects are sensuously similar. This is why X-rated movies and even visually stimulating love stories are so popular; they can simulate the feelings and even the sensations of the actual experience. The body cannot distinguish between the physical and the mental; between what is actually occurring in our life and what is being imagined with our mind. If our body can get turned on when we are consumed with thoughts of sexiness, what happens when we are consumed with thoughts of sickness? For those who are scientifically, left brain minded, research has proven how a thought affects every cell of the body right down to the DNA. For those of us who are not scientifically minded, watching how the ease or dis-ease of our mind instantly creates the same in our body is about the best research we could ever ask for.

Just a passing thought?

Are we now supposed to become paranoid about every so called negative thought that we have? Of course not, that would defeat the whole purpose. We are working to become more at ease with ourselves and our life. The purpose is to show that if there is a dis-ease in the body, from a major problem to a nagging headache, to a lack of ease, energy and exuberance, we can be sure that there is a corresponding dis-ease within. To lose sight of that principle or to argue that the ache, pain or ill came from some outside source puts us right back in a defenseless and dependent position. If we deny the connection within for the physical dis-ease, blaming everything from germs to government, then we also deny the creative power to heal it. If we abdicate our own power, believe that something or someone outside of us has caused the problem, then we must rely on something or someone outside of us to fix it. As we take an honest look at the success of that approach to health, relying on anyone and everyone to fix us now and 'insure' us for the future, we just might have some second thoughts. The constant aches, pains, chronic ills and rampant fears about illness that beset almost every-one, ourselves included, plus the obvious rarity of radiant, fully functional healthy people as examples around us, give us a current diagnosis and a future prognosis that if we stick with only the tradi-tional physical approach to health, conditions can only get worse. However, untraditionally speaking, we are predisposed, that is naturally inclined to be well, really well. In fact, it has taken quite a lot of 'B.S.' to pull us off that path. It won't take but a small effort to get back on the path, the path of natural healing.

There are countless books and tapes illustrating real life stories of people who have healed their outer dis-eases, from chronic to ter-minal ones by healing their inner dis-eases. Dr. Bernie Siegel wrote in his book, *Peace, Love and Healing*[7], over 90% of people who have recovered from 'incurable' illness will tell you about a signifi-cant change in their life prior to the healing. An existential shift has

---

7   Peace, Love and Healing, Bernie Siegel, M.D.

occurred in them and for the first time in their lives they are truly living. Other people's stories greatly help dispel the doubt about our own healing power and reinforce our right to releasing it, but no one else's story proves the principle quite like our own. Instead of relying on the American Medical Journal for our answers, it is time we start our own real life journal.

Healthy mind. . . more than a good cliché

The phrase *healthy mind/healthy body* is as common today as physical fitness. However, the phrase healthy mind is far too often just an *adjective* instead of an action *verb*. It describes a certain state of mind, vague as it may be (what does a 'healthy mind' really mean?), but how to get to this state leaves many people dumbfounded. Certainly focusing on dis-ease - from a cold to a cancer - does not lead to a healthy state of mind. But, as we have seen, the mind is not just a source of thoughts, it is also a source of feelings. These feelings, even those that bypass our awareness, have a major effect on the body. To believe that we can have radiant health or even freedom from illnesses without healing the mind as a whole, particularly things that are bothering us, has been one of our major downfalls. Even the most avid health fanatics, those who watch every morsel of food that they eat, exercise religiously and stay far away from any unnatural or toxic substance, are kidding themselves if they ignore the longings and grievings of their own mind. No matter how well we eat, it is not until we get to what is eating us that the real healing begins. Fortunately, this is an age where getting in touch with our feelings is not only acceptable, it is encouraged. Getting in touch with what is bothering us is a major step.

The Botherhood of man

There is a long-standing aim of mankind, an idea that returns generation after generation and that is the 'brotherhood of man'.

Although strides have definitely been made in that direction, we still seem to be far from harmony. Maybe we have been missing a step that comes before the *brother*hood of man called the *bother*hood of man. As has been evidenced by the less than ideal results over time, it is impossible to have harmony in the *world* if we do not possess that harmony within ourselves. Unfortunately, this principle has been widely accepted, even used as inspirational material but *accepted* and *practiced* are very different things. If we want to see everyone as our 'brothers', we need to clean out much of what 'bothers' us about our brother. As many of us know, what bothers us about others or life in general had to be *in* us to be stirred by *any*one else. Even if we are not really concerned right now about furthering the brotherhood of man, we still need to find out what bothers us if we are concerned about furthering our health. There is a direct connection between what is bothering us in our body and what is bothering us in our mind. Heal the latter and the former automatically returns to health. Heal the *former*, however, and the latter will come through in another time and place. With these temporary results, why *bother?*

Again there is good news and bad news to healing our 'bothers' and ultimately, our body. The good news is that once we get in touch with what bothers us, an amazing change takes over in our body. It seems like the vises that were tightening our muscles are loosened. If we really do *feel* what we are feeling, a relaxation comes over us that in comparison, makes us realize how tight we were. Symptoms like a headache, stuffed nose, pain in the stomach or anywhere in the body subside. And if we make peace with the 'bothers', in addition to the wonderful ease, a renewed sense of energy and enthusiasm begins to flow.

The bad news is that we may have become such a master at repressing, denying and hiding our feelings - good and bad - that they are removed from our consciousness before we can say "something's bothering me." Once however, we decide that we want to touch the hurt, feel the anger and connect with the fear, we are far less bothered by what had seemed painful before. The real pain was not in the feeling but in the fighting the feeling. As we get in tune with what bothers us, as we give up the fight, we are finally free.

Actually, *we* cannot truly heal the mind anymore than *we* can heal the body. There is only one healing power and no 'one' nor any 'thing' can ever duplicate it. Our job is to find a way to allow it to finally flow. Healing works the same for the mind as it does for the body. As we continually and consistently remove the inner blocks (the 'B.S.'), both the mind and body are healed. The healing power can only do *its* job when we do *ours.*

The healing of feelings

There are many excellent theories on why people must live on the surface of their minds, trying desperately to avoid any deep feelings, negative *or* positive. For one thing, we are led to believe that emotions, especially if they make us feel vulnerable, are the warning signs of instability and childishness, in a word, bad. If we cry, show anger, express deep fear, admit guilt, then society labels us and these *natural* emotions as abnormal. Showing great joy, although infinitely more healing, loses out to being sturdy and in control. Even letting go with full hearty laughter is frowned upon. Somewhere in the early years of our childhood, feelings that were expressed uninhibitedly, got shot down. Well meaning parents, teachers and other authority figures, in an attempt to teach us 'good behavior' told us that it is better to *act* good than to *feel* good. Very early on, we learned to bury, hide or manipulate any strong feelings in an effort to appear mature and steady. But this definition of maturity, acting stable on the outside while avoiding the war on the inside renders the longed for state of inner peace impossible. As long as the war rages within, our body will continue to bear the battle scars.

An 'alternative' to Alternative

It is good, really good that we have so many alternatives to traditional medical care. "Alternative Health" or "Alternative Medicine"
have become new systems of healing; from biofeedback to acu-
puncture and dozens of new ones every year, their purpose is to
avoid making the treatment more harmful than the illness. And to
this end, they are a blessing. Whether they should always be chosen
over traditional medicine depends of many factors, none of which
we are here to debate. But if we believe that alternative systems
are truly wholistic, we will fall into the same hole as we did with
traditional medical care. Most alternative practices, while far less
toxic and far less traumatic than traditional practices and in many
cases, highly successful, lack the vital principle of true healing.
They are for the most part, done *to* the person, whether that be *to*
the mind or *to* the body. The benefit slowly wanes when the treatment is over. True healing means a lasting change has been made
and cannot be attained by doing something *to* a person, but rather
eliciting something *from* them. Even the most natural of treatments
are still for the purpose of curing *illness,* leaving the path of *creating health* yet untrodden. Availing ourselves of these alternative
methods when we are ill rather than being stuck with only medical
treatments is a whole lot better place to be, but it is *not* wholistic.
There is more to life and more to health than having *less* problems.
A wholistic life, no less than wholistic health is about connecting
with our higher self. And for those who want more life and health
more abundantly, there *are* no alternatives.

United we stand, divided we fall

The divided or conflicted mind, one that has compartments of acceptable feelings and those that are unacceptable or wrong, is the
main destroyer of wholeness. The erroneous belief of today is that
we should *think more* and *feel less;* 'B.S.' Actually it is impossible
to separate our thoughts from our feelings - we think with who we
are - but the effort we make to separate our thoughts from of

feelings kills any chance for holistic healing. Although holistic or wholistic healing has been used to describe everything from cholesterol to colonics, its true nature is far more than physical. Wholeness, by definition, means *free of injury, free of wound, undivided, unbroken, unmodified, physically, mentally and spiritually sound, complete, in its entirety, a person in his full nature without any exception, total, full, without separations.* Instead of being divided, broken and split inside, as is too often the norm, becoming more whole is more appropriate and allows *all* feelings to flow freely. The lack of wholeness on the inside, resulting in the lack of health on the outside, is not about the *nature* of our feelings as much as it is about the *barrier* to them. A divided mind, like a divided nation, will destroy itself. We can still try to blame germs, government and God, but it is the dis-ease within the divided camps of feelings that break down the body and the life. This is good news, once again. If it is the dis-ease that *causes* the problems, from failing health to failing marriages, then ease is the *cure.* Allowing our feelings to surface, wanting to touch the 'untouchable' hurt, pain, anger as well as longed for love and joy, begins us on the path of true peace. It is only from this point of peace or ease that both happiness and health can be created. There are no exceptions to this rule. On the other hand, becoming united, connected and joining with our feelings as a whole creates a security and strength that stands through any adversity and heals any ill.

Trying to fix the problems of the body or our life by the outside only - physical treatments, drugs, herbal therapy, getting the approval of others - only pushes us further from our purpose of wholeness. But even if we think that wholeness can wait, and that a healthy, illness free body is enough, we are falling into the same holes. Healing is a whole or nothing approach; it takes the power of the spiritual to heal the physical. And when we talk about healing, we don't mean fixing one ill or one crisis after another. True healing raises the body and the being to a whole other level where health is elevated, not just illness eliminated. And to think that we have been led to believe that health and healing is *from* the body.

The quiet mind

Talking about a 'healthy mind' is today's normal approach to this inner healing; *working* toward it everyday is the natural approach. So what can we do on a regular basis to come back to a whole, healthy mind? Daily quiet time, meditation or self reflection is the first step. Before starting our day or just before going to bed are the best times to re-center. This need not be anything formal, a quiet place with a comfortable chair is enough. We can close our eyes and let our mind drift as we did in the R-I-D-E exercise. This time, however, you are acting *before* there is a problem, true preventative health. The goal is to allow our mind to do its thing, unravel as it will and heal as it needs to. This may result in a frantic scramble of thoughts; what happened, what we have to do that day, or some unresolved feelings. That is the mind's way of clearing without the noise of our thinking that occurs relentlessly during normal business hours. After days or weeks of doing this quiet time on a regular basis, we will notice some periods of real ease. From that calmer mind, and *only* from that mind, the healing power can flow through the body with great magnitude. Health, from that quiet state, will take on a whole new dimension.

Hasn't it always been this way?

Conditioning, (a milder term for brainwashing or mind control), is how society draws its adherents. Whether it is for the sale of a product (how can anyone live without a VCR or PC?) or blind belief in an approach (vaccinations fall under this 'never ask why' condition), conditioning makes us believe it always was and always will be. It has been only about ten years since recycling went into effect in each state. We used to throw all garbage in one bag; now we would feel like a criminal if a glass bottle slipped into our regular garbage.

Talk about how conditioning can make our minds putty in the hands of advertisers and authorities; the whole attitude toward

smoking has made a 360 turn. Anyone over the age of 30 may remember when smoking was still a rather 'cool' thing to do. Now it
is not only 'uncool' but smokers are given the cold shoulder by almost every nonsmoker. Watching the smoking attitude on old
black and white movies and TV sitcoms is almost impossible to
comprehend if you were brought up with the Belief System since
the early 1970's that smoking is the cause of so many horrendous
dis-eases. Lucy and Ricky lit up everywhere with no problem, in
fact, it was a socially accepted grace. With today's promotion of
'second hand smoke,' *second* looks are proceeded by *dirty* looks.
We are not here to debate the right or wrong of smoking; to do that
and be fair, we would have to look at all the anger and fear *about*
cigarettes as well as the nicotine *in* cigarettes.

Vaccinations fall under this 'never say why' conditioning. The results of blindly following this 'standard procedure' without investi-
gating the negative side effects have been toxic and fatal. The
reason that we care to approach such volatile subjects is to show
how conditioned we can and have become. The danger of conditioning makes us react before we think; in fact, we believe that we
have thought about the issue, when in reality, we have been *thought
for*. We have been so conditioned to respond to a certain stimulus,
(like Pavlov's dogs who salivate every time they heard the bell), that
good, healthy, logical judgment gets run over by mass belief. This
is especially true when fear is part of the condition process. Kids
are often led off track by *peer pressure*; adults succumb instead to
fear pressure. And nothing is more conditioning or fear pressuring
than today's shoot in the arm, shove it down the throat answers to
our health problems. Conditioning at its best, but gaining any access to our healing potential at its worst. As we become less conditioned and more creative, (the purpose of this book), healing hits an
all time high.

Sharing our wholeness with the world?

"How are you," is the most common or rather conditioned questions in the English language. The question stimulates responses like, "I'm doing OK; I got a nice raise." "Pretty good, my husband and I are taking a vacation next month." "Not that good, my bursitis is acting up again."

What would happen if we answered that question from a 'whole' new angle? "I'm doing OK; I think I just got in touch with a major anger in my mind that has been draining me for years." "Not bad, I feel myself getting more balanced and dis-ease free within." "Actually I am a bit concerned about how divided I feel inside and how I keep avoiding certain painful feelings." "So much better since I began connecting with my higher self." Unless a person were involved in a wholistic healing program themselves or had a few too many wine coolers, these answers would alienate the best of friends. And yet, answers like these, reflecting our inner rather than outer conditions, are not only more accurate but more effective. Perhaps in the year 2000, everyday conversations will take on this 'whole' new quality, but until then, let's walk it more than talk it. Living as a whole person will speak for itself. It is ironic that the majority of people are quite open to discussing their outer dis-eases and the latest cause and cure (shellfish?) but when it comes to inner dis-eases, they all clam up. Wholistic healing need not win a popularity contest to work for us. What this higher aspect of health has lost in mass appeal, it has more than made up for in mass abundance for those who use it.

Mental wholeness

There is no exact formula for healing the holes of dis-ease in our mind and becoming whole again. Each person will need to find their own system over the days, months and years ahead of working on themselves. Fortunately we will have the rest of our lives to perfect it, as inner healing must be constant if it is to really heal.

We no longer need to wait until we are *sick* (even in mind) to get *well*.

Stimuli are everywhere and often it seems that 'bad things happen to good people,' but no circumstance justifies a dis-eased mind. Whether people or situations wronged us is not the issue here. Healing conflicts in our life come down to choices and as far as gradually attaining a dis-ease free and radiantly healthy body, there is only one choice. The conflicts, stress and pain in our *head* must be resolved if we are ever to see the resolution in our *body*.

The objective observer

Separating ourselves from our feelings without running away from them is quite a step toward inner healing. For so long we *were* the feeling, if we *felt* hurt, we *became* the hurt, or we did everything possible to avoid it. As we enter the realm of inner healing, as soon as we sense disturbance, something 'bothers' us, the goal is to objectively and intimately observe it. We need to *reveal* it, then *feel* it and finally *heal* it. Instead of taking life so personally, (feeling like everything is happening *to* us, as an objective observer we take life more spiritually, looking at what is happening *through* us. As soon as even a twinge of unsettledness occurs, we observe it, find out what it is, get in full touch with it, then work to get back in ease once again. Taking a R-I-D-E with our feelings (instead of feeling *driven* by them), is an excellent exercise to reunite with ease.

A whole new way of being

From this day on, let us exercise our right, our birthright, to mental and physical wholeness. Let us vow each day to become more and more connected to what is happening on the inside, both positive and negative; to heal the holes and feelings that are stimulated so often. From this process of mental wholeness, staying connected with *all* of our feelings, true inner freedom begins. The process of freeing our minds of the thoughts that so long have disturbed us, releases the flow of energy that has been blocked; energy that can now heal our chronic pain and ills. When mental resistance begins to disappear (flowing with life and our most uncomfortable inner feelings), the walls of discontent and dis-ease begin to melt. Getting above our own thoughts where we can watch the disturbance without becoming disturbed, begins true healing.

This process of restoring our wholeness is a lifetime goal. As we begin to objectively observe our everyday thoughts, particularly those that irritate us, surface disturbances begin to heal. As these surface ones are eased out, deeper more profound disturbances and dis-eases will become clearer. As we reveal fear and heal the real sources of hurt, anger and self pain, health and life are elevated beyond belief.

As the surface disturbances ease - irritations with our boss, worry over money, wounded feelings when a loved one doesn't appreciate us, minor self criticisms when we make a mistake, the healing can deepen. Now the fun begins. Although it is difficult to see at first glance, many times we immerse ourselves in the same surface problems day after day to divert our attention from the deeper ones. But there is more to pain than meets the surface eye; and the 'warning signs' are every place. Being irritated or annoyed with our boss usually indicates a deeper anger and resentment buried within us. Worry over money may well indicate deeper fear that quietly haunts us all the time. Wounded feelings tend to indicate a deeper hurt that has never been faced. Minor self criticisms, where we half jokingly put ourselves down, usually indicate deeper guilt over not being the good person we thought we were supposed to be. Self criticism is also indicative of the profound self rejection that has punctured a hole in the very heart of our being.

Resentment, fear, hurt, guilt, self-criticism and disillusionment are the holes in which our wholeness, our joyful inner and outer flow, gets totally drained. In fact, it is these deeper unhealed feelings that cause the real pain in our body and our life. The real tragedy is not these feelings (they can be healed), but the blame that we place on the outer world for stimulating them in us. As long as we believe that someone or something is responsible for our resentment, fear, hurt, guilt, self-criticism or disillusionment, we build barriers to healing greater than the Berlin Wall, barriers that no drug can heal. We may have been led to believe, as they had in Russia, that a wall protects us against enemies and pain, but the opposite is really true. Walls block healing and love even more than they block enemies and pain. The walls that we build to protect us from our own painful feelings are the 'soul' reasons that we feel deeply unloved and stay unhealed. On the other hand, as we welcome with open hearts these previously banned, deeper feelings and sincerely work to let them go, the pain within and without like the Berlin Wall, begin to crumble.

Turning our backwards approach to healing 'inside out'

As the principle of mind/body oneness is observed more in our life, as we see how a *new* image or a release of an *old* hurt literally transforms the physical body (right down to the DNA), we will feel greatly at ease. The fear of illness that drained the life force out of us has begun to slip away. At the same time, the joy of radiant health is slipping in. This whole new state of being assumes that we are actually living the principles of mind/body oneness. This means we make sure that thoughts, images and feelings of the mind are in conformity (instead of contradiction), to what we want in the body. As we work more from the mind, we will just naturally move away from the backwards, totally physical approach that believes healing comes *from* the body.

The world can continue to poke, prod, puncture and 'pill' the body for another millennium, but we can choose another way. We may look like we are from another planet when we no longer try to get healed *from* the body, but the tables are turning. As more and more people raise their level of health by raising their approach, those who ignore the mind will be looked at as out of their minds.

Getting in the spirit of healing

How many times have we heard the defense, excuse or insecurity, "My mind just isn't strong enough to heal my condition"? Whether this response is an avoidance tactic or a real fear, it shows another misunderstanding regarding health and healing. While healing is not from the *body*, technically or spiritually speaking, neither is it from the *mind*. Healing flows *through* the mind and is transformed by ease or dis-ease therein, but to say that it is a mental process puts the burden of healing back on our shoulders. Healing is a spiritual process. A process that is higher and deeper than any of us can imagine. If we still are having a hard time budging from the one dimensional mechanistic approach - the pill theory - this spiritual concept of healing may be a bit 'hard to swallow'. By this point, however, we should be finding the pill theory a bit hard to swallow.

Once we realize that healing is the very nature of the universe, as well as the very nature of our own being, we will then throw out the 'pill theory' as the long awaited 'cure-all'. Does this mean that we throw out all our pills and refuse to consider them in our health plan? Not necessarily. The traditional medical approach to health can still be used to *assist* our healing but it cannot or should not be used as a substitute for the real source of healing.

Daily, regardless of the current health of our body, the spirit of healing needs to be foremost in our minds. When confusion and fear over health set in, let's consider the source, the source of our confusion and fear (the 'B.S.' that sickness is a 'normal' part of life), and the source of healing, (the ever flowing, unlimited in its power, spiritual dimension of healing.)

The separation of church and state ·

When did it happen? When did we choose the path of machine
over mind, the path of statistics over spirit? Somewhere along the
line as a society, our senses became so dazzled by the phenomena
of medical science that we lost sight of the healing power of our
own being. This focus on external things and the disdain for anything that sensed of God or the spiritual, especially regarding
health, probably began with the separation of Church and State
which commenced its untying in the 1500's. It is certainly true that
no organization, church or government should control our choices.
Certainly, centuries ago, the church did unfairly and fearfully domi-
nate the minds of the people. But to eliminate all that religion or
more appropriately, spirituality has to offer because of this problem
is cutting off our nose to spite our 'faith'. Further, to believe that
spirituality connecting with the Divine power within and without
has no place in everyday life is the 'B.S.' underlying every problem
today, health being no exception. The cure for our suffering, the
answers to our prayers, are in the higher dimensions of our being.

This separation of the spiritual and the physical is in good part responsible for our dilemma in health today. To limit our health to
what we can physically do *to* the body and ignore what comes spiritually *through* the body, leaves us totally dependent on someone or
something else to keep us well. In a way, we are right back to the
days of church domination, only this time our leaders work from a
laboratory instead of a pulpit.

To ease some of the fears surrounding spirituality, know that it
need not be anything formal or religious. Plato, the prominent
Greek philosopher, long before the time of organized religion
preached the word of wholistic health from a spiritual level. His famous quote, the great problem with health today is that we try to
separate the soul from the body is as true now as it was then. Because of our paralyzing fear of dis-ease and our deportation of the
spiritual realm back to religion, the inner part of us has been

tragically neglected. It has taken a thousand years or more to realize that Plato, without a single American Medical Association Journal knew the secret to health.

Is it really necessary to understand the 'whole' picture of healing?
Couldn't we just do the 'mind' thing and call it a day? Not really,
we would 'love the faith' and get swallowed up by the old fears of
illness somewhere along the way. However, when we understand
what Jesus meant when he said, "it is not I but the Father within
that doeth the work," we always know where to turn. The Father
within, the Power within, God, the Spirit or any name that we
choose to call this higher aspect of healing matters little. What
matters is that we know that this healing is constantly available to
us anytime and all the time and not just *waiting* but *wanting* to flow
through our being. Knowing that there is a healing spirit that is
greater than any problem in our body can finally put our mind at
ease.

Healing. . . no longer just 'for' the body

There is no question that society's obsession with the body has gotten out of hand. Wiping out all the major illnesses we currently
have in the world seems to be the most crucial goal of the day. Although one doesn't need a crystal ball to predict the likelihood of
this happening in the near future; the number of ways the body can
breakdown has been increasing every year. Think about it, even if a
dis-ease free world were in the cards for us, some very profound
questions must be asked; "Would we finally be *happy*? Would we
have found *peace*? Maybe we need to first find out whether health
problems are the *cause* of our unhappiness and lack of peace, (as is
the prevailing belief), or is our unhappiness and lack of peace the
cause of our *health problems*? Do the things in life (from health to
wealth) bring us the happiness and peace or does the happiness and
peace bring us the things in life? Jesus had a simple answer to these
profound questions. He said, "Seek ye first the spiritual (the higher

ideals of life) and all else will follow. It seems that we need to look at the healthy life concept from a 'whole' different angle.

There is no question that living without illness, not to mention living without the fear of illness, would add much to our life. But eliminating physical ills from our life is not the answer to ultimate happiness, it isn't even the answer to ultimate *health*. True health, the health that we were meant to have, only *starts* at the body; a dis-ease free and radiantly healthy body is only the physical dimension of our health. Being truly healthy means that we are as spiritually well as we are physically well. The spiritual dimension of our being is the most valuable to our health plan and yet too often the least valued. (Do any of us belong to a Health Plan the covers us for spiritual well being?)

The minor emphasis placed on evolving spiritually is due to the misconception (more 'B.S.') made about the real purpose of life. The 'normal' view is that we are physical beings given a spiritual dimension to evolve more *physically*. The 'natural' view is that we are spiritual beings given a physical dimension to grow more *spiritually*. With the 'normal' view has come all the normal problems, anxiety, pain, worry, lack, conflicts with people and ever growing illness with spurts of happiness, security and health. The 'natural' view brought by Plato, Jesus, Moses, Emerson and all the great minds past and present bring a sense of joy, peace, security with the universe as well as physical well being. The masters all knew that true health is as much a security with the universe as it is a wellness with the body; it is spiritual at least as much as it is physical. Now we can see why society's take on holistic health - vitamins, nutrition therapy, homeopathic remedies, massage - are all valuable but they are not spiritual. We need to nourish our spirit with at least as much enthusiasm as we nourish our body and concern ourselves with what is toxic to our spirit even more than with what is toxic to our body. Then and only then the truth of 'wholistic' health as well as the higher purpose of our being is served.

The 'wholeness clause' written into the contract of life

It is not uncommon to think, "Isn't all the spiritual stuff a lot to ask? Don't we have enough stress, problems and work in our life?" Maybe we need to consider the fact that there would be far less stress, problems and work in our life if we 'sought first the spiritual.' Seeking first the physical sure hasn't given us the peace, health, wealth and ease to which we are Divinely entitled, but each of us must come to that conclusion ourselves.

But Nature is no fool. To prevent us from focusing only on these outer riches at the expense of our inner riches, she instilled in us a 'wholeness clause'. There can be no true satisfaction on any level until we open up to all levels. Nature uses our body and its diseases to aid our inner growth. The 'B.S.' that our body gets ill as a punishment or because of some unrelated, meaningless cause is a gross religious and cultural misunderstanding. The body as well as all areas of our external life serve as a printout of our mental and spiritual state of being. Dis-ease - pain, difficulty and discomfort - in our body and in our life signals us to a dis-ease on the inside where the suffering is really most profound. Physical ills, from a pain in the neck to a pain in the heart are our cue to stop and find a way to return to mental and spiritual ease. It sounds strange to the ears of traditional health proponents, but physical ills can be our greatest teachers and greatest healers. Once we realize the indisputable wholeness clause that is part of our human makeup, we will look at the body and all physical aspects of our life as the path, not the problem, the gage not the goal. From this perspective, the richness to our life is limitless and compounded daily.

Does this mean that we have to get physically ill to get spiritually well? Not necessarily. We certainly don't need to bang into the back end of a truck to know we are driving too close. If we keep our eyes on the road, watch what is going on in front of us, as well as what has happened behind us, the ride can be smooth and accident free. It is the same with the path of our being. If we keep our eyes on the road of life, watch our body and external life for signals of where to turn within as well as healing the beliefs of the past, the ride can be smooth and dis-ease free. That is how human life was intended to be. But just in case we decide to get off the beaten track, Nature put in a fail safe. Dis-ease of all kinds are meant to stop us in our tracks and get us back on the road to inner and outer bliss. External dis-ease and pain automatically heal when we heal internally and evolve spiritually; in fact this is the only way. We can't fool Mother Nature. With the rewards of following her plan, why would we want to?

Toxic today. . . nourishing tomorrow

It seems society is 'health' bent on finding the *things* that poison our body and the *things* that cure it. The problem with the *thing theory* is that everyday the things change; what was toxic last year is benign this year and vice versa! It is hard to remember what has been 'pulled from the shelves' so to speak and what is back in circulation. Do cellular phones still contribute to cancer? How can we ever feel secure with a system that is never constant? We can't. As long as what is toxic and what is nourishing remain on our 'to do' and 'not to do' list, (primarily physical), we will miss the whole point of healing. Healing is about the whole being and cutting caffeine or eating more fiber does little to raise our spirits. The physical 'do's and don'ts' are important, but to do or not to do is a small piece of the whole pie.

'To be or not to be', that is the question

Except for an occasional reference to stress or relaxation, the dozens of lists of what is good for our health and what is bad for our health rarely touch the realm of *being*. What we are doing for our health has its merits but whatever we are *being*, the core of ease and dis-ease within, overpowers anything on the physical realm. This is why it is all too common to find people who, according to the current 'do's and don'ts', do all the right things but still suffer with health problems and can't figure out why. Solicitous to a fault in their 'healthy' lifestyle, these people fervently deny themselves anything that even looks like it could be unhealthy. They wouldn't smoke if their life depended on it; in fact they are well versed on the negative effects of 'second hand smoke'. We should be so well versed on the 'smoke within'. Not discounting the toxicity of nicotine, a change needs to be made in our health priorities. Before ranting and raving about the negative effects of 'second hand smoke', we would be wise to check out the effects of 'first hand resentment.'

There is more to healing than meets the mind

Just like a dis-ease in the body indicates a deeper dis-ease in the mind, a dis-ease in the mind indicates a deeper dis-ease in the spirit or inner self. We may be bothered by the world outside of us; people may irritate us, conditions may worry us and circumstances may disillusion us. But there is more to these feelings than meet the mind. As we break down the mental dis-ease of the moment, allow it to reveal what is really bothering us, we may find unresolved dis-ease that has been with us for a lifetime. Core fears, guilt, hurts, grievances and self-rejection from past situations or with life in general are the source of the uneasiness or dis-ease we feel on a daily basis, whether we are aware of it or not. We may have unknowingly chosen to anesthetize ourselves from our self, keeping far away from the deeper issues, but the effects still rage on. For healing to be complete on the physical part of our being, it needs to eventually (the sooner the better), be completed on the spiritual. Questions like "What am I really so *fearful* of? What am I so *guilty* about? What am I so *hurt* about? What *grievances* am I still holding on to? Where did all this self-rejection come from?" should be asked. Questions about profound dis-ease should however be asked from a point of profound ease, if possible. No matter what is going on externally or even internally, a source of unlimited, unchangeable and unconditional power is always behind it all. As much as is Divinely possible, let us see our dis-ease from the eyes of the ultimate Healer.

What is behind it all?

So is this the whole purpose of our existence, to unceasingly unravel the pain until either we or it become totally unraveled? No. We are not a pain looking to heal. We are a healing looking to flow, a Divine healing. Getting in touch with the deeper pain and dis-ease is monumentally freeing. In fact we will never know true freedom until these core issues are touched and resolved. But behind it all, behind the so called dis-ease (maybe it is just deeper dimensions of our being needing no positive or negative label), is the real Power. Perhaps it can't even be said that this Power, this Universal Divine Energy is *behind* it all. Maybe this higher dimension is really *through* it all. Maybe that is what is meant by being truly 'whole'; we can't define where the pain ends and the power begins. Maybe it is all one in the end. If this is true, as has been said by the greatest minds of history and still being proclaimed today, then we are not really working to heal the pain, but to feel the Power.

Since we are filled with this Power, this Divine Intelligence or God (if that suits us better), then blocking the pain also blocks the power. We cannot get around it; behind it, or through it, this Power is one with all our feelings. Denying one, we deny it all; feeling one we feel it all. The choice is certainly ours to make, but when it comes to true wholistic healing and Divine living, do we really have a choice?

What's the point?

We could do it. With enough time, energy and belief, we could get the conditions in our life to be exactly how we would want them, for a period of time, anyway. And certainly a healthy, abundant life is more than within our right and ability; we are a child not a *stepchild* of God and the universe. But as Jesus said, "What would it profit a man to gain the whole word and lose his own soul?" or to paraphrase, what is the point of being settled physically and unsettled spiritually? From guilt of the past, emptiness in the present and fear about the future, these spiritually unhealed feelings dull even the best of times. Our search for happiness, peace and security (the main needs of our inner nature and the 'warning signs' of true health), are not as has been advertised, the by products of the products that we buy. In fact, the more immersed and obsessed that we are in the physical dimension of life (from wanting it to worrying about it), the less connected and open we can be to the spiritual dimension. "Ye cannot serve two masters." And it is in the spiritual that the true peace is found, regardless of whether or not all the pieces of our life are together.

The beauty of the spiritual nature is that it does not depend on our physical state of being; our life can be upside down but if we are focused in the right direction, our spirit can be complete and together. As soon as we raise our consciousness by filling it with more spiritual ideals, the fear, guilt and emptiness that keep us from truly enjoying life (and we thought it was our lack of things) are no longer there. It is in the state of consciousness; the spiritual ideals from which we base our life, that our physical life is created.

Being filled with a sense of joy, free from fear and worry and unmistakably tranquil in *any* circumstance of our life, it is this state of consciousness that lifts *all* the circumstances of our life to a richer state. As long as we are continuously healing our *inner* nature (feeling and resolving what bothers us), and ever growing toward our higher nature (filling ourselves with spiritual knowledge and regularly meditating on our Divine connectedness), we are getting "life more abundantly."

True healing. . . for the whole of us

True wholistic health is no longer something we *do,* it is something we *are.* More accurately, it is no longer for our body but for ourselves as a whole being. It may seem that this kind of life takes an awful lot of work, in the beginning, like any new venture, it will. From our experience, however, as well as the words of all the great minds past and present, the effort put forth in this kind of healing is nothing compared to its rewards; the return is a hundredfold. We feel as though we have just begun this journey toward discovering the divine purpose in our life and are able to put some of it into practice, even though we have been studying for many years. Yet even using just some of these principles, our health and our world has been dramatically enriched. Are there still aches, pains, stresses, problems? Of course. But they are less, less often and less painful. Yes, it feels at times like we are traveling across the wilderness in a stagecoach pulled by intoxicated horses journeying into unknown lands. But *always* some unseen force, some inner power is right there to help us along the path. That is the Divine Promise to every being who "seeks ye first the spiritual." There has never been a single moment of regret on this journey, no matter how often we get sidetracked or stuck. On the contrary, each day brings with it an excitement about going further. As Stymie from the Little Rascals said while speeding down the hill on a self made jalopy, "I don't know where I'm going, but I'm on my way!" We are all like Stymie, we are not totally sure where we are going but we know that we're on our way!

The end of the 'B.S.'

It has been quite a journey getting through society's Belief Systems on health. The truth of how much 'B.S.' has been fed into our mind about the limitations of our body can be overwhelming at first. Fortunately, we are overwhelmed now to avoid being overtaken by the 'B.S.' later. We found out that whether or not an idea is actually true is immaterial, if we *believe* it to be true, it determines the material aspect of our life, health being no exception. And once we accept an idea as true, whether it is really 'B.S.' or not, we make it our foundation and build other ideas upon it. In essence, we may have built 'B.S.' on top of 'B.S.' which is what Part I of this book has been about.

The first of society's 'B.S.' laid the foundation for all the rest. **'B.S.' # 1: Health is the exception to the rule** taught that we can create the life that we want in any area *except* health. This is such a universally accepted 'B.S.', at least in the western world that few people even attempt to create a new image and level of health. This means that the old image of health, one that is generally filled with fear, warning signs of illness and belief in chronic pain will keep creating the same old health conditions. And with the direction that society is going in regard to promoting 'health' (more and more ills to come), our old health image can only get worse. From this point, believing that we have little if any creative control over health, that health is a process of luck rather than logic, leads to the acceptance of the rest of society's 'B.S.'

'B.S.' # 2: Someone else *can* and *should* take responsibility for our health builds upon the first 'B.S.' If we have no creative control over our heath, what would be the point of taking responsibility for it? From all we've learned in 'B.S.' # 2, creating the state of inner ease from which health will then flow is only able to be done by us, so we must assume responsibility. Can it still make sense to wait for a pill or a treatment to be 'discovered' that will do for *us* what we know can only be done by *us*? If we still believe that an outer system, (Health insurance, the Health Care System), can do more than our own inner system, then we will 'wait versus create' and hope 'they find a cure.' Unfortunately, that approach is not only irresponsible it is impossible; sad to say to many, it is still logical.

Now, if we deny taking responsibility for creating the mental ease that leads to physical ease, it would not make much sense to create the mental picture of the health that we desire. We would then be satisfied with living by **'B.S.' # 3: Good health means not being sick.** As society parades before us the growing number of illnesses right in our midst, the new flu coming our way, or another drug for the neverending headaches, backaches and allergies suffered by almost everyone, or the pill to clear up your indigestion so you can still eat all the junk food you want, (remember, you can't fool mother nature), the sick image is pretty clearly laid out for us. If we listen to the 'B.S.', we are destined to believe that *not being sick* is another name for *good health*. To make matters worse, our idea of 'not sick' may be sicker than we thought. In our fear of becoming *dysfunctional* with a serious ill, we as a society have accepted *functional* health - on again off again aches and pains, occasional bouts of illness, constant tight neck, back and shoulders - as good enough. With this standard of 'good health', *fully functional* health, our natural state, is rarely if ever a normal thought.

Living with an image of health being 'not that bad' but not all that good does not lend itself to a wholistic ideal. If anything, this leads us more toward **'B.S.' # 4: Healing is *from* the body and *for* the body;** we will be more inclined to focus all our energy on the body. This focus will lead us to try inducing healing *from* the body, through some drug or physical treatment, (even if 'all natural'). Logic might inspire us to think that if there could be a cure created, it would have been created by now. But there is a second part to this fourth 'B.S.', the belief that healing is *for* the body (only) and after all isn't that where all society's efforts are placed, leaving us with a major hole in our wholistic needs. Ignoring our mental and spiritual needs for healing is just the ignorant attitude that has left health in our country in such a sick state. Healing is of the spiritual, even if we are talking about healing the physical; it comes from a much higher dimension than any physical 'thing', our body included. Healing is also *for* the spiritual as well as *from* the spiritual. Opening up to and growing toward the Divinity within us; working to purify our nature, (at least as much as we work to purify our nutrition), is what true healing is all about. Anything less is just 'B.S.'

PART II:

Beyond our Personal Belief Systems 'B.S.' about Health

Thank God for this 'New Age.' The movement toward fully functional, radiant health has given our society a much needed sense of hope and purpose. We have, however, only just begun. Although this genre of thinking is as old as the hills, the actual 'practice' of it, at least in the Western world, is in its infancy.

When it comes to creating a truly healthy life, just reading about the principle of mind over matter or studying wholistic health pursuits that seem so profound is only the first step. Unfortunately this intelligent rhetoric has up until now been the whole of our practice, leaving us with a lot more knowledge but little more health.

The reason that wholistic health has yet to be accepted as a valid system is not because its 'effectiveness' is inconclusive; the healing power within works 100% of the time. The tentative results are because our proper 'use' of this power is inconclusive; we talk it more than we walk it. Fortunately, things are changing. . .

Seeing perhaps for the first time society's 'B.S.' was the beginning of this whole new level of health. Part II takes a more 'personal' turn. Our personal beliefs, responsible for much of our chronic aches, pains and ills, are finally brought to light in this section. Getting beyond our personal 'B.S.' can miraculously heal in 'no time' the problems that would have undoubtedly endured a 'lifetime.'

Getting personal

Part I of this book was devoted to the general 'B.S.' about health and sickness that plague us all. Part II gets a bit more personal. Once we heal the foundation of our health ideas as in Part I, we are clearer to get to the individual beliefs responsible for our individual health issues. And if we were shocked at some of the 'B.S.' in our head on a *general* level, the *specifics* will really hit home. Of course, the more up close and personal they get, the more healing will be ours. This is exactly what happens anytime any of us transgress our beliefs, health being no exception. The problem with health as opposed to religion is that we are usually unaware of our own beliefs, especially those of a personal nature. Part II is the beginning of our personal awareness.

The system that will be presented in this section works; any system that opens us up to the healing power within will work, this one being no exception. So many people have told us that this system has lessened if not eliminated chronic aches, pains and health problems that previously were glued to them. Nothing feels quite as wonderful as being free of life draining pain, no matter how slight; in fact we may be surprised how slight it *wasn't* once we are free of it. Personally, we are quite grateful to this system for easing up *our* gnawing pains, what's more, the healing keeps unfolding as we get closer to our innermost selves. This neverending healing is just waiting to flow for everyone and there is no exceptions to this rule.

Part II reveals and works to heal each of our most 'personal' h • .lth 'B.S.' To successfully reveal and heal these beliefs, they will be presented in four different exercises corresponding to the four Personal Belief Systems. The exercises are in order of the depth and the subtlety of the 'B.S.' Each successive exercise will be subtler and more potent than the last. The following are the four beliefs and exercises:

Exercise # 1: General 'B.S.' about Health
Exercise # 2: Metaphors of Life to Health
Exercise # 3: Sick Benefits
Exercise # 4: Sick and Tired of the 'B.S.'

Our thoughts and speech are so habitual, so normal that we are not
always aware of what we are thinking or saying. Where were we
taught the art of conscious awareness; objectively observing what is
going on in our minds and what comes out of our mouths? Until
perhaps reading this book, we may never have tried to connect the
manifestations in our body and our life with the thoughts and words
that preceded them. How often the answer to a problem is right
under our nose, but we can't or maybe *won't* see it. "I'm not angry
in the least," we say with smoke coming out of our ears. "I believe
I can be radiantly healthy," we declare, not two minutes after wondering if the stiffness in our neck will ever go away.

The point is not to *fix* our beliefs (only to have them return) but to
free them permanently. Many of these beliefs have been with us for
years, so they are not clearly apparent at first. As we read and do
the following four exercises, allow each and every belief some time
to whirl around in the mind before accepting or denying it. Some
beliefs are so 'matter of fact' that it will take a little time before we
realize how profoundly they have been running or *ruining* our
health.

Not always seen by the naked mind

We have already pointed out that it is much easier to *stay* well than
to *get* well, to build upon an already positive dimension of health
than to try and pull ourselves up when our body is filled with pain
and our mind with panic. There is, however, something to be
gained from the pain or the panic. It is at this point that our real
beliefs come screaming to the surface. Sure we can rattle on about

the glories of radiant health, the magic of the mind and the unlimitedness of the healing power within when we are feeling *good*. Until we dedicate our life to watching our thoughts and beliefs *all* the time, catching the most subtle ones, we will need a jostling experience or a surge of fear to make us conscious of what has been driving us subconsciously. What happens when a symptom pops up in our body from a common sneeze to an unusual bump? Where do our thoughts go when things are not going so well? Does fear, worry or a mental image of our body going downhill become uppermost in our minds? Do we then concentrate or frequently think about the symptoms and the impending ill or pain? Or on the other hand, does our mind remain steady with an image of a healthy body? Instead of panic, do we see an unlimited power flowing through us, bringing healing to wherever it is needed. Do we maintain a picture of radiant health even when our body does not seem to be the 'picture of health?'

Unless we have made a conscious study of our own beliefs, it will take time and awareness before we can see them as they really are; deep beliefs cannot always be seen by the 'naked mind.' The following four exercises will help accelerate the process of awareness. If we choose to be open and honest with each question or point, a real belief will surface. By now, we probably realize that there is more then a little 'B.S.' standing between us and greater ease, energy and exuberance. At this point in the book, there is no need to 'B.S.' ourselves into believing that our health problems, current or future, come to us from some outside source. If they came *upon* us, they were created *within* us. And that truth is the most beneficent, God given principle that we have; if we created the problem, we are just as powerfully endowed to create the solution.

An exercise in humility

This first exercise deals with the most common 'B.S.' about health; they are generally accepted but individually selected. They are shared by almost every one in our society; in fact you can hear a conversation going on reinforcing a particular one of these beliefs everyday. It is suggested to read each one carefully and take several seconds to see if that particular 'B.S.' holds any truth in our life, checking or highlighting those that do. Remember, this is not a test. There are no 'right' answers. It requires humility to get past the 'B.S.' and not deny or defend a belief just because it is ours.

Revealing the 'B.S.'

By this point, especially after reading and intensely analyzing society's beliefs in Part I, many of the statements in the following exercise may not seem like 'B.S.', the fact is they are *all* 'B.S'. In other words, the twenty statements, although accepted as facts by most 'learned' of people, are all learned beliefs. Each one, when accepted as fact, lead us and our body to the corresponding result. If for example, we take # 5 as a fact, then we will probably be one of the many 'flu sufferers' each year. If we *don't* take # 5 as a fact, then we will most likely *not* suffer with the flu even when all around us everyone is sneezing and wheezing. We can argue that physical conditions - germs, weather, nutrition, body chemistry, etc. - cause our physical conditions and they do *affect* these conditions, but bottomline, it is our beliefs that 'clinch the deal.'

It is true that many people would rather put time and energy into defending the physical cause of their ill than to work at changing the belief, but that choice should be old news to us. We should be getting to the point of *discovering* our beliefs rather than *defending* them. Discovering our beliefs is a delicate process; they are subtle and tricky. To really heal the 'B.S.' in Exercise # 1, it is suggested to go over each of the twenty points again and check off those, perhaps missed the first time, that even slightly tug at us.

Exercise #1: General 'B.S.' about health

[ ] 1. Worrying about health is normal and natural, even preventative.

[ ] 2. A chronic condition is difficult if not impossible to eliminate.

[ ] 3. It is normal and natural to get at least one cold per year.

[ ] 4. There is little one can do to prevent certain conditions, illnesses or viruses.

[ ] 5. During 'flu season', it is likely to get the flu.

[ ] 6. There is little one can do to stop allergies during 'allergy season.

[ ] 7. Headaches, backaches, stomach problems, sinus problems or other annoying but non-serious ills are a normal and natural part of life.

[ ] 8. Illness is unfortunately a normal and natural part of life.

[ ] 9. When ill or in pain, it is difficult if not impossible to stop thinking or worrying about it.

[ ] 10. If we have a problem with our body then we are sick.

[ ] 11. The likelihood of the body breaking down increases with age.

[ ] 12. Certain health problems are likely to happen at certain ages. (at 35, this can happen, at 40 this. . .)

[ ] 13. If someone is sick at home or work, it is very possible that we will 'catch it.'

[ ] 14. Some illnesses or chronic conditions are more difficult to heal than others.

[ ] 15. Worrying about the health or illness of a friend or loved one is normal and natural, even caring.

[ ] 16. A pain or symptom in our body is cause for concern and/or worry.

[ ] 17. Change of weather, drafts, going our with a wet head are likely to get us sick.

[ ] 18. The mind/body connection works with some conditions but not with others.

[ ] 19. Illness is something to be feared if not very concerned about.

[ ] 20. Healing comes from 'health experts'.

Healing the 'B.S.'

Now that we have *revealed*, it is time that we *healed* the 'B.S.'
Both processes are ongoing throughout the experiences of our life;
more of these and other beliefs will be revealed now that we are
looking for them. As we find them, we will continue to heal them.
For now, look at the points in Exercise # 1 that were checked off as
our beliefs. Look at the words that are underlined in each point.
They are the key words underlying some of the major reasons that
our body breaks down or chronically hurts. With all that has been
learned from Part I of the book, logically reason on these beliefs.
Gently, but firmly think about why these beliefs are really *not* facts.
Choose words and ideas that contradict the 'B.S.' For example, if
we previously believed that chronic conditions are difficult if not
impossible to heal, (#14) we can heal this by saying something like,
"Anything can be healed with the unlimited power within. I see
myself with less and less of this (condition) everyday. Do this with
all those that were checked. Take enough time with each one until
the 'B.S.' even feels like 'B.S.' to us. Remember, a few minutes now
can save us weeks of illness and pain later. The revealing and healing will still go on after this exercise. In fact, the underlined words
will help us remember it is only 'B.S.' When the thought or fear
pops into our minds as the days go on, being aware that it is 'B.S.'
will prevent it from overwhelming us.

If you still have doubt, we refer you to take a course in Concept-
Therapy[8] or read any of Dr. Deepak Chopra's books on health.
This following excerpt from The Rhythms of Life[9], proves that our
body, and every system in it, is unceasingly renewed every day, every month, every year. For example,

[8] CTI, 25550 Boerne Stage Rd, San Antonio, TX , 1-800-531-5628
[9] Smithsonian Institute, Washington, DC, 202-357-1300, Crown Publishers 1981

from *Rhythms of Life:*

Area of Body	Cell Renewal
Lining of the mouth	Every 5 days
Stomach	Every 2 days
Colon	Every 4 days
Skin	Every 308 hours

Logically therefore, if the body continually and naturally reproduces new cells of each tissue, organ and system, how then could any condition be truly chronic or unchangeable? Could a so-called chronic condition really be a result of our *chronic beliefs?* And remember, if there is just one person who can reverse a certain condition, or one person who doesn't get sick during flu season, it is possible for any of us.

Reinforcing the foundation

As we begin this 'personal' healing, remember the principles discussed in Part I. Part I laid the foundation for our health from this point on; we can never review and reinforce these principles enough. This foundation also allows for the personal transformations that are presented in Part II. Let's review the principles from Part I: (1) Health is as much in our creative control as any other goal in life. (2) It is our privilege and our responsibility (we have both the choice and the power) to create the health we desire. (3) Radiant, fully functional health - ease, energy and exuberance - is our new standard of 'good health.' (4) The physical, mental and spiritual aspects of our being as a whole are the unlimited resources from which anything is possible. Being in tune with this creative power can heal anything physical as well as strengthen our Divine connectedness.

Keeping these ideals fully alive in our minds we can finally get beyond the 'B.S.' that has kept our health so limited. Keeping this in mind, go back over Exercise # 1 one more time. The unlimited power of the universe is at our direction; knowing that should render the belief that a cold, flu or allergy can overcome this immutable force illogical, if not totally 'B.S.'

Metaphysical to 'better physical' health

When Louise Hay's first books, *You can Heal your Life* and *Heal your Body*[10], were published in the late '70's, their metaphysical and metaphorical suggestions created quite a stir. These books proved from countless real life experiences that our body directly and quite literally reflects our inner feelings. Ms. Hay contends that certain thoughts such as fear of accepting joy or constant self criticism will manifest in specific dis-eases, like high cholesterol or frequent headaches. Her books have been a tremendous help to us with our own personal health quest as well as in our consulting with so many others. We have found Ms. Hay's metaphysical and metaphorical diagnosis's to be right on the money.

In the 1980's, the decade of 'health and fitness,' talking in such metaphysical or metaphorical terms when related to health and illness was kept to private groups. Believing that our body tried to communicate to us through the symbols of illness was at that time, analogous to believing in extraterrestrial beings. In the late 1980's we tried to explain to a close friend who knew by heart the warning signs of every major ill, that her chronic cold sores may be due to her 'fear of expressing the angry words she was thinking', from Louise Hay's *Heal your Body*. Her cold sores should have healed right then and there after the angry words she expressed at us for the "ridiculous and insulting" analysis. Although it almost ended her friendship with us, something must have hit home. Today, she and her family are great supporters of wholistic and natural health. In fact she often tries to 'metaphysically diagnose' her friends and family, often receiving just about the same reaction she gave us in the late '80's. But several of her friends and family have also been bitten by the 'holistic health bug', taking a natural and inner

---

10   Louise Hay, Hay House, P.O. Box 6204, Carson, CA 90749-6204

approach to health. Fortunately as we approach the 21st century, metaphysical practices are 'out of the closet.'

It is no longer blasphemous to suggest that someone other than a 'real doctor' can be a healer. Releasing the healing power within is not limited to a person with a medical degree. A person with a 'degree of peace' can enjoy the most remarkable health.

True 'body language'

When our body is dis-eased, a dis-ease within us is directly or indirectly responsible. The lack of *ease* in our body is a signal of a lack of ease in our mind; in other words something is in conflict within us.

The body is a symbol for our thoughts and feelings. It speaks to us in a language that everyone understands, the universal language of pain. The faster we become aware of the message, the less the body needs to broadcast the pain. (That is the purpose of the exercises in Part II). To still doubt or dispute this truth means only that we have not yet agreed to check it out in our own life. Once we become aware of the hidden fear, unhealed anger, self abasement, guilt, gnawing hurt and/or creative frustrations with our job or our relationships and work to reveal and heal these feelings, it is impossible to deny the corresponding flow of ease in our body. The focus here is not on *what* is expressing in the body, but *why*.

Exercise #2: Metaphors of Life to Health

[ ]   1. This is such a <u>headache</u> for me.
[ ]   2. I just <u>can't</u> *look* at this.
[ ]   3. I <u>can't see</u> how this will ever work.
[ ]   4. I will just have to <u>grit my teeth</u> and bear it.
[ ]   5. When will I learn to keep my <u>mouth shut?</u>
[ ]   6. I <u>can't talk</u> about it.
[ ]   7. I just <u>can't face</u> this right now.
[ ]   8. I'm <u>pulling my hair out</u> over this.
[ ]   9. The words just get <u>stuck in my throat.</u>
[ ] 10. I <u>refuse to swallow</u> my pride for anyone.
[ ] 11. I just <u>don't want to hear</u> that anymore.
[ ] 12. He is such a <u>pain in the neck.</u>
[ ] 13. I <u>refuse to stick my neck out</u> ever again.
[ ] 14. Why is everything always <u>on my shoulders?</u>
[ ] 15. I feel like <u>screaming my lungs out.</u>
[ ] 16. I have so much to do I can <u>hardly breathe.</u>
[ ] 17. This is weighing <u>heavy on my chest.</u>
[ ] 18. My <u>heart aches</u> with such sadness.
[ ] 19. I was so nervous I almost had a <u>heart attack.</u>
[ ] 20. I <u>can't stomach this</u> anymore.
[ ] 21. You make me <u>sick to my stomach.</u>
[ ] 22. I wish everyone would just <u>get off my back.</u>
[ ] 23. I have no <u>backbone.</u>
[ ] 24. I am <u>weary to the bone.</u>
[ ] 25. I <u>don't have a leg to stand on.</u>
[ ] 26. I just <u>can't walk away</u> from this.
[ ] 27. I have <u>one foot in and one foot out.</u>
[ ] 28. I could just <u>kick myself for that.</u>
[ ] 29. That makes my <u>blood boil.</u>
[ ] 30. The <u>pressure is killing me.</u>
[ ] 31. I <u>refuse to bend</u> on this one.
[ ] 32. I am so <u>tired</u> of this.
[ ] 33. I get <u>hurt so easily.</u>
[ ] 34. What a <u>sick world</u> we live in.

This exercise connects clichés that we use on a daily basis, often unconsciously, with the metaphoric reflections in the body. Although we would be amazed at how often we say and think these phrases, they may seem a bit foreign to us at first glance. Rest assured that during any given heated discussion or complaint, one or more of these metaphors pop up. Follow the same directions as with the first exercise; read each phrase carefully and think about it for a few seconds. Check or highlight those that are said or thought on a regular basis.

It is hard enough on our health when we are *generically* upset, but using our body to describe how upset we really are, just compounds the effects. It has been well proven that the mind and body are connected, if not one in the same thing. Knowing that fact makes it even more dangerous to use negative health images, like headache, tired or pain in the neck to describe our feelings. The mind grabs on to the most powerful idea in a sentence (our real feeling) and does its best to translate it into the body. If we want to feel more energy and exuberance in our body, saying that we feel like the 'weight of the world is on our shoulders' does little to support our goal. And once again, it is our responsibility to fill our being with the image that we want for our body.

Review those metaphors in Exercise # 2 that were checked off. The words underlined are the underlying ideas that may be negatively affecting our health. From now on, be aware of saying or thinking these negative ideas and stop the cycle. Refuse ideas that are not of a healing nature. Practice everyday saying and thinking *healthy* metaphors. "My life is exuberant." "I am so energetic." "The healing power flows through me easily, clearly and effortlessly." Our body and life are a literal transcript of our innermost ideas. Why would we choose those that literally and metaphorically make us sick?

The cliché of clichés, the metaphor of metaphors

For years we have been fascinated by the connection between a person's inner and outer worlds, particularly when it comes to health. Clichés/metaphors hold such interest as the translation to the body is uncanny. While a whole host of clichés and metaphors make up our daily consciousness, there is one that sums up all of them. How often do we hear the clichés/metaphor *sick and tired?*

If there is one phrase that serves as a catchall for both our inner and outer dis-eases, it is *sick and tired.* Not only does it accurately symbolize the inner frustration, ("I'm so sick and tired of these money problems"), that seems to permeate most waking hours, but it personifies all too perfectly the physical effects in our world; how many people do we know, possibly ourselves, who are frequently *sick* or chronically *tired?*

If we are not yet able to realize how often that we ourselves say or think the sick and tired phrase, we cannot miss it in any normal conversation. Whenever anyone is angry, disgusted, stressed or feeling taking advantage of, there is a good chance that this cliché will assert itself. "I am sick and tired of being treated this way." "I am sick and tired of all the pressure." "I am sick and tired of never having enough money." The problem once again is not in the cliché, but in the lack of conscious awareness. Are we fully aware of the situations, people and aspects of our life that we say we feel so "sick and tired" of?

Sick and tired of the denial

In a society where 'positive thinking,' putting on a good face and emotional control at any cost are the standard to which we aspire, taking responsibility for feelings of frustration or pain may seem like admitting defeat. Of course everyone admits to 'stress', it has

become the socially acceptable aphorism for life. In fact many people like to brag about the amount of stress they have as though it is
synonymous with importance or too many things to do. But admitting to stress rarely heals the inner pain. For one thing, stress is
generally thought of as *someone else's fault.* We are stressed because of our job, the economy gives us stress, our in-laws, spouse
or kids stress us out. So we put the responsibility for our feelings
on someone else, which is an impossibility. The second reason that
admitting to stress does little to heal the inner pain is that it has become a universal dumping ground for all frustrations. Whenever
we feel uptight, it is 'stress.' This catchall phrase dilutes and denies
the real feeling, keeping this real feeling far from our conscious
awareness. So instead of getting to what we really feel, the only
way healing ever takes place), we dump any negative feeling into
the stress file. But "be not deceived," as Jesus said, "God is not
mocked; whatsoever a man soweth, (thinks in his heart), that shall
he also reap, (manifest in his life)." We can call it stress or even a
negative attitude, but until we admit to being deeply frustrated,
highly disappointed, greatly hurt, intensely angry, extremely self
guilty or profoundly scared, the 'stress' lives on.

Like the *functional* state of health, we can become comfortable
with minor discomforts when it comes to stress. Waking up and
going through most of our day with a *fair amount of stress* is not
only normal in today's run, run, run world, it is deemed inevitable.
This bit of trivia comes from the same philosophy that claims a *fair
amount of health problems* are inevitable. We, of course, know
now how limited that kind of thinking really is. We were born with
the potential for unlimited health and we were born with the potential for unlimited happiness; in actuality, we were born with the potential to be *unlimited* in every area of our life! So to believe that
stress, even a little is normal and natural is just more of the 'B.S.' to
which our society has become accustomed. Ease of mind, (the opposite of stress), feeling free, calm and happy is not only our privilege, it is once again our responsibility. It is our 'real job' in life.
More to the purpose of this book, living with stress means living

without **Health beyond Belief.** There is no half and half course. When we are *dis-eased* in mind, even a little, we are *dis-eased* in body. But beyond the effects on our body, who wants to live with a constant supply of stress flowing through our being. Aren't we 'sick and tired' of the stress already?

Sick and tired of the stress

Nothing causes more stress in our being than feeling 'sick and tired' of something, someone, some condition or some feeling. Being 'sick and tired', a phrase that is emphatically used and quite literally translates to our body means that we have not made peace or come to *ease* with a thing, person, condition or feeling. In other words, it has *stressed us out* for far too long. The day in day out or even every so often run ins with these particular situations are wearing us out, inwardly as well as outwardly. But if we are so 'sick and tired' of being 'sick and tired', why don't we do something about it? For one thing we are generally unaware, at least consciously, of the many situations of which we are so 'sick and tired'; we have unfortunately become quite used to them. For another, even if we *are* aware of them, we believe that they cannot be changed. 'B.S.'! With a true awareness of what we are really 'sick and tired' of and a change in thought *about* these situations, anything can be changed. Furthermore, our health literally depends on it. Nothing can make our body more 'sick and tired' then being 'sick and tired' of our life. And contrary to popular 'B.S.', admitting to a feeling does not make it *real*, it finally allows our being to *heal*. Exercise # 3: Sick and Tired begins this healing.

In as honest and open a way as possible, knowing that this exercise begins healing some of the deepest and deadliest of stresses, we need to ask ourselves "what am I most 'sick and tired' of in my life or my head?" It can be things, people, conditions or inner feelings. Part A deal with external situations. Part B deals with internal and more personal situations. After thinking a few moments, fill in the blanks.

Exercise # 3: Sick and tired

A. "Sick and Tired" of the physical situations in my life, (family life, money, other people, conditions.)

(1) I am 'sick and tired' of _____
because he/she/it makes me feel:

_____

(2) I am 'sick and tired' of _____
because he/she/it makes me feel:

_____

(3) I am 'sick and tired' of _____
because he/she/it makes me feel:

_____

B. "Sick and Tired" of the emotional or self limiting situations in my life (health, weight, abilities, self worth, feelings.)

(1) I am 'sick and tired' of my _____
because it makes me feel:

_____

(2) I am 'sick and tired' of my _____
because it makes me feel:

_____

(3) I am 'sick and tired' of my _____
because it makes me feel:

_____

No matter how often we do this exercise in our workshops, people are always amazed at how 'sick and tired' of life our whole society has become. This phrase is thought or said many more times than most of us are aware; this exercise brings more of that awareness to light. Besides being unaware of how often we relate to this phrase, many are unaware of how much this phrase relates to our body, no less our whole being. If we feel 'sick and tired', - run down and exhausted, less than motivated, generally have the 'blahs' - anywhere in our being, this phrase may be the culprit. And anything that we are 'sick and tired' of, because of its relentless, neverending nature, drains our whole sense of self. That is why we add to the exercise how it makes us feel. In truth, how it makes us feel is the real core of our being 'sick and tired.'

Sick and tired of negating our feelings

The more we realize that we are meant to live a healthy, joyful and peaceful life, the more 'sick and tired' we will be of feeling 'sick and tired.' The stress that this vicious cycle puts on our body is surpassed only by the stress it puts on our joy for life. The treacherous part of this whole situation is that it has become so normal to be 'sick and tired' that it takes an exercise like this along with a vow to carefully watch what makes us 'sick and tired', before they get a chance to rear their ugly tired heads. True to its nature, this 'B.S.' is subtle and sneaks up on us when we are not observing.

From 'sick and tired' to healthy and alive

Before we become 'sick and tired' of this whole idea because it does require some thinking, there is good news. No matter how damaging it has been up until now, if it is 'B.S.', it can be healed. First, we have to become aware of what we are 'sick and tired' of. Second, we need to go back over the 'sick and tired' responses and heal them; we have no choice if we want to be healthy and happy. The choices that we have are to either do something about the situation, (which we have not done or have been putting off), or we have to make peace with the situation as it is. Choosing the latter means that we really work on the feeling until the *dis-ease* is gone and only an *ease* remains anytime the situation crops up again. Although the process may take days, weeks or months to actually see the healing, the shift occurs in the mind immediately.

As far as how each 'sick and tired' makes us feel, that is an issue unto it 'self.' The situations which we are 'sick and tired' of make us feel angry, *scared, unloved, hurt, worthless, pressured, like a fool, taken advantage of, like things will never change or only get worse,* (if ideas like these were not part of our answers, we may want to think about whether they should be.) Regardless of the verbiage used, it all translates to a 'self' issue. Something within or about our self got rocked; either it was a self worth issue or a life worth issue. Either way, it hit a belief we have about how we feel as a person or a belief about what we can have in this life. Whichever it is, it is something *in* us that got stimulated by something or someone *outside* of us. If it is in us, it is our responsibility to heal it. What we have learned up till now in these chapters about our Divine birthright for unlimitedness will be a big help. Part IV, *Self Healing*, will also add greatly to the healing of our 'self'.

We don't have to be sick anymore

There is nothing more sickening or more tiring than going around the same circle with the same 'B.S.' day after day, year after year. In reality, nothing that happens to us is all that frustrating in and of itself. What kills our spirit and our will is when we see no way out, or forfeit our ability to change. While we are "sick and tired" of many feelings, believing that the 'B.S.' we are going through is a life sentence or that it will never change is devastating. Feeling that we have little or no control hits every system of the body, particularly the immune system like a nuclear explosion. But it is probably beginning to dawn on us that the victim role is a choice, not a curse. Waiting to heal that which we are 'sick and tired' of (the money problems, the relationship conflicts, the weight anxieties, the low self worth), and the negative way it makes us feel (angry, scared, taken advantage of, hurt), can really heal our life as a whole. Whether we are doing something physically to change the situation or we have decided to accept it with ease as it is, there must be a change in thought and feeling (a change in consciousness), for true healing to take place. When the consciousness has changed, when we think and feel differently than before, when a new picture of the old situation is created in our minds, when a degree of *ease* replaces the terminal *dis-ease* in our mind from before, then change takes place everywhere. Many times this change of attitude or conscious- ness eventually turns the whole 'sick' situation around. Taking back the power, reclaiming our victorious role in this universe, (if Dr. Frankl could do it in *his* situation, it is certainly possible to do it in *ours*) changes our previous 'sick and tired' foundation of life to one of 'radiant and alive'. Using terms like these instead of the 'sick and tired' ones, is the last step in healing.

Taking a proactive role in our health to evolve physically, mentally and spiritually as a natural course has not been the norm. Up until now, waiting until there is a health problem, usually one that is seri- ous or dysfunctioning to our life has been the best stimulus for change. It is true that physical *dis-ease* can be our greatest wake up call, especially when we have ignored the mental and spiritual *dis-ease* that always precedes it, but this is the hardest place from which to work. We are weakest and least hopeful about making a life enriching change when we are sick. At that point the only thing on our minds is to get rid of the pain in our body. But given a short period of time, the pain, sometimes with a new face and label comes back; technically it never left!

Sick benefits

When Doreen told people that she was hired right out of college by one of the largest 'health' corporations in the world, almost every- one had the same comment. "They've got great benefits." Being truly naive, she figured the benefits were something like trips to the

Bahamas, frequent galas or special gifts for doing a good job. When the advantages of working for such a prestigious company were explained, instead of the glorious trips, elegant affairs or wonderful gifts, the primary 'benefit' was that no matter how sick she got, it would be *fully covered*! Doreen felt like a kid in a candy store who just discovered the sweetest treat was chocolate covered spinach. As the Personnel Director of this major 'health' corporation went down the list of drugs, treatments, surgeries and complete round the clock care should it be needed, she found herself feeling a little queasy. He further explained that if she became incapacitated due to a major accident or a serious illness, it would be covered with their excellent disability package. Was this a joke? Was somebody really filming her expression to send to America's Funniest Home Videos? The little blue booklet entitled, "Sick Benefits" made Doreen realize that this was no laughing matter. Being the optimist she is however, Doreen said to the Director, "Well you explained all the advantages of working here and getting *sick*. What are the benefits for working here and staying *well*?" He looked at her as if now *she* was the one making a joke.

That was fifteen years ago. Corporate Health Care has changed in one sense and remained the same in another. It is no longer free, (employees now share part of the cost), but the 'benefits' are about the same. Companies still try to woo prospective employees with sick promises; how ill they and their families can get and how much these ills will be covered. Even if they intensely dislike the company or the work that they do, many people choose to work for a certain company or refuse to leave their current job because the sick benefits are just too good. We are not debating the necessity of health care insurance any more than the necessity of car insurance; at this point in our evolution we need it. But to buy a car, one that we intensely dislike driving just because we get good coverage is ridiculous. Why then do we accept working at a job where we are unhappy just because we get good coverage, (especially when our job unhappiness is a major contributor to the breakdown of our health). We can of course change our attitude about our job; if we cannot do the work that we love, we can always love the work that we do. But there is another choice as well. As we realize the truth that as long as we work to create health daily, radiant health will be our natural state. With this principle to back us up, we can choose a job that will fulfill our potential talents, not our potential hospital stays.

We can joke about the paradox of corporate 'health' benefits; that it focuses on how *sick* we and our family can get and how much is covered under the company 'Health Plan'. Yes, they are necessary but the health care systems, both in the corporate world and in society provide little incentive for staying well; most alternative methods (non-invasive, more natural) as well as preventative approaches (exercise programs, mind/body health workshops, books/tapes), are rarely covered. As it stands right now, the Health Care System continually impresses upon us, indirect as it may be, the subtle benefits for being sick. It is shocking when we first realize that there are *professional benefits* for being sick. The real shock comes however, when we become aware of the *personal benefits* for being sick.

The real 'sick benefits'

Oh boy, this is a tough subject! Explaining how each of us may unconsciously *benefit* from being sick, that in the dark recesses of our being, we *enjoy* being sick and may unknowingly work to *create* a problem in our body, is to some about as insulting as it gets. That is why we saved this provocative principle for the end of Part II. Do we still get looks of *how dare you!* when we introduce this idea in our workshops? All the time. But so far no one has maintained their look of insult after this subject has been fully explained. In fact, many have felt that much of their suffering was directly connected to these 'sick benefits'. (Even with the miraculous changes that we have seen, we have deemed it wise not to tell the general public that they may be getting a rise out of being sick!)

No miracle drug, no ingenious treatment and no all-inclusive health coverage can make but a dent in our health as long as we retain some personal benefit for being sick. That is a fact, although many would claim that having a personal benefit for being sick is just plain 'B.S.' It is 'B.S.', but 'B.S.' when accepted as truth influences our life just as much as tr·+h does. "Whatever a man soweth, that shall he also reap", works on whatever the idea is, whether we have consciously chosen the idea or not. 'Sick benefits' fall into this category. None of us would *consciously* choose to be sick. . . or would we?

The fine line between consciousness and conscious choice

At one time or another we have often wondered why friends or loved ones keep putting themselves into the same negative situation over and over. If it is depression, we may wonder, "Do they *like* being miserable?" If it has to do with negative relationships, we may think "Maybe they *like* being mistreated." If a person keeps overeating even though they know the effects, we may consider, "I guess they *like* being overweight." Unless there is a solid trust between us and the person in the negative situation, it is safer to keep these thoughts to ourselves. If however, these thoughts cause us to think, "Do I *like* suffering with the things that keep happening to me?" then, this negative observation can have some positive effects.

It is true that on some level we have chosen the feelings, situations and effects in our life, (what a man soweth. . .), health being no exception. But to say that we *consciously* chose to suffer, that we *like* having problems in our life would be a hard concept to grasp. Actually, we *do* create the self, the health and the life which we are now experiencing, but there is a gentler, more logical way of expressing this truth. The less than desirable conditions in our self, health and life are more a matter of conscious*ness* than conscious *choice*. Something within us is in direct harmony with the conditions or feelings that we are experiencing; it cannot happen any other way. The 'something within us' however, is not always as plain as the nose on our face. The inner beliefs that attract or create the outer feelings and conditions are universal, we *all* have them, but they are highly personal, even private. So they remain buried and hidden, even from our own awareness, where they continue to attract or create the same negative experiences again and again. But for those who want to end this cycle, the 'B.S.' stops here.

Benefits that are hazardous to our health

Contrary to the normal mode of thinking, positive goals of health, love and success are not always positive to *us*. Until we reveal and heal our limiting beliefs, some of the best things in life can fill us with the worst of feelings. Negative feelings such as unworthiness, fear of failure, even fear of success, are often riled when we try to make positive changes in our life. Conversely, seemingly positive feelings like getting attention from others, release from responsibilities, even atonement for guilt often result from the most negative of situations; sickness being the most common. This paradox of negative feelings for positive results and positive feelings for negative results, if not understood, can sabotage the goals that we try to attain, especially in health. More people are ill, suffer for an entire lifetime with chronic aches, pains and ills or forfeit their right to radiant health, because of this idea of 'sick benefits' than from all the caffeine, nicotine and cholesterol put together.

Of all the personal 'B.S.' discussed so far, the benefits that we get for being sick or in pain are the most potent and the most difficult to see. It will take further time and self observation after this exercise to see the actual connection between the benefit and the breakdown of the body. For now and for this exercise, check off the subtle desires that have been quietly burning a hole in our mind. As per each of the previous exercises, read each point slowly, then deeply think whether it strikes a cord. Part A of Sick Benefits gives us a one liner of desire. Part B explains the desire in more vivid detail. The more insidious our desires/sick benefits, the more likely that they will be hidden from our sight in Part A, but more likely to hit us between the eyes in Part B.

Exercise # 4: Sick Benefits - Part A

[ ] 1. desire for *attention or love*

[ ] 2. desire to <u>stop living for other's approval</u> and expectations

[ ] 3. desire to be *free from self pain* for failing to achieve our goals or standards

[ ] 4. desire to stay in bed, or <u>do something just for us</u>

[ ] 5. desire to be *left alone*

[ ] 6. desire to *avoid confrontation* with some person or situation

[ ] 7. desire to <u>get away from daily grind</u>

[ ] 8. desire to be <u>free from burdensome responsibilities</u>

[ ] 9. desire to take on <u>others' sufferings</u>

[ ] 10. desire to be <u>free from guilt</u> for causing hurt or not giving enough to others

[ ] 11. desire to <u>atone</u> for sins and wrongdoings

Exercise # 4: Sick Benefits - Part B

[ ] 1. <u>A desire for attention or love</u>: Unable or reluctant to ask for the attention that we need and want when things are going well. Get most attention and sympathy when sick or in pain. Hard to accept love or express hurt feelings *except* when sick.

[ ] 2. A desire to <u>stop living for others' approval and expectations</u>: Even if never told so, often feel like we have been a disappointment to others, haven't lived up to what we think others expect. Always feel we should do or be *more*.

[ ] 3. A desire to be *free from self pain* for failing to achieve own goals or standards: Rarely satisfied with accomplishments or feel 'good enough.' Feelings of failure or unmet standards haunt us often.

[ ] 4. A desire to stay in bed, or <u>do something just for us</u>: Never feel we have enough time for us. Dream about staying in bed, relaxing, watching TV or doing something fun, something that we love to do but never feel we *could* or *should.*

[ ] 5. A desire to be <u>left alone</u>: Often feel pulled by or from pressure or depended on by others - boss, coworkers, mate, friends, family, etc. - and wish we could be left alone for a while, often feel smothered.

[ ] 6. A desire to <u>avoid confrontation with some person or situation</u>: Try to avoid confrontation - arguments, intimidating people, uncomfortable situations as often as possible. Procrastinate in making decisions because of fear of making a 'wrong' decision.

[ ] **7. A desire to get away from daily grind:** Often feel trapped, unhappy or bored with daily activities. Wish we could change our life or at least escape for a while, but deep down see no way out.

[ ] **8. A desire to be free from burdensome responsibilities:** Often feel stressed and burdened by some or all of our responsibilities. We feel a sense of anxiety or worry most of the time, thinking that we cannot do all that is demanded of us.

[ ] **9. A need to take on *others sufferings*:** Often suffer with the pain, problems of others, whether it is someone we know or just hear about. Tend to feel guilty if someone else is suffering and we are feeling good.

[ ] **10. A desire to be free from guilt for causing hurt or not giving enough:** Feel a constant gnawing that have done something wrong or not done enough of something right; never good enough. Take personal blame for mistakes, mishaps and problems; always hard on self when something goes 'wrong.' Frequently worry that have hurt, offended or disappointed others. Rarely compliment self for the good done or said.

[ ] **11. An ongoing need to *atone* for sins / wrongdoings:** Often harsh, critical, condemning with self, especially when we do 'wrong.' Feel constant need to atone - to be either punished or forgiven - for faults, mistakes, self inadequacies. Belief in self suffering, even a little.

The mind's wish is the body's command

The basic principle of energy is that it can either be moved or
changed; created or destroyed is not an option. Beliefs, thoughts,
feelings are like everything in the universe; another form of energy.
And since energy cannot be created or destroyed, whatever is going
on in the mind (the energy) is not just going to disappear. It will do
the 'energy thing' and translate itself into the physical equivalent the
best that it can. Desires to get attention that is received during
times of sickness or pain, desires for justifications for not living up
to our own or other's standards, desires to get away from the daily
grind, or relentless burdens, desires to take on other's sufferings,
not to mention desires to atone for sins, usually through some form
of pain or punishment must be expressed into their physical coun-
terparts. Chronic health problems, muscle aches or physical pain
have become the most common 'attention getters', excuses for not
doing what is expected, ways to escape from it all, as well as the
path to self punishment; pain in any form usually is.

Doreen had a self defeating 'disabling' experience at her first job
with that major health corporation. She viewed her situation with
the accounting work as being trapped with no way out, dreading
the beginning of each work day. She remembers often dreaming of
saying good-bye to the job without having to say good-bye to a
salary. One day while driving home from work her dream came
true in a manner of speaking. She had a serious car accident. Unfortunately the disability ended sooner than the pain from her inju-
ries. There certainly could have been a 'healthier' way to move on.
Most people would laugh at the insinuation that Doreen with her
God given creative power attracted the 'accident'; after all it was an
accident! But she knows better. Not five minutes before she
crashed, the remembers clearly thinking "I just can't face another
day at that job; she never did.

Pat had a similar run in with the 'law' (of the universe), that is. In
the early days of their business switch from exercise to researching

wholistic health, money was low and need for approval of their talents was high. Their first major client satisfied both needs, though his morals were questionable. Pat and Doreen knew he was dishonest but they ignored this 'minor' flaw and freely took the money, so they thought. After a few months of taking the money and running, they began to run into their own guilt and disgust. They were doing a job for which they were overpaid and taking money from a man they didn't like or trust, (so who was being dishonest?) Pat was the one who actually took the money and ran; she picked up the check every two weeks. On her way to get the check one Friday afternoon, Pat left the office disgusted and ashamed for selling her soul for a weekly paycheck. She felt that she could not go on like this one more day. She, like Doreen, was in a major car accident soon after she reached the 'breaking point', a point that nearly broke her. Thank goodness it was only a great wake up call. The contract with the three shady characters, (Pat, Doreen and the client) ended the next day.

Does the body have to be the punching bag for the mind's desires? Yes and no. Yes, if our desires go unheard and unhealed. No, if we choose to reconcile them. Go back over the checked desires, (making sure to review the *unchecked* ones for a missing connection), and choose a method of healing. Either physically *do* something positive that will fulfill the desire, or change the attitude that created the desire in the first place. Perhaps what we think others' expect of us, our own standards, what is really burdening us or the guilt over our mistakes haunt us more than we ever realized. If they are, which is most likely the case, then an honest, supportive, hope inspiring talk with ourselves or someone who we trust can release the pain behind the desire. As can be expected, once the inner pain is gone, there is no longer a 'benefit' for the outer one.

Sick benefits. . . a twisted kind of logic

If we believe the inner pain is more fearful, shameful or painful than anything that could happen outwardly, then we will unconsciously create *anything* to avoid dealing with it; health problems being far from the exception to this rule. In a twisted, macabre way, therefore, outer problems, especially pain and sickness, actually become 'benefits'. They universally excuse us from all the self created *shoulds and shouldn'ts* in our life. Guilt, rejection and lack of love are to many, far more painful than any outer ill. In addition, sickness and pain have become society's platform for compassion; when we are ill, all bets are off. We are given the love, forgiveness, kindness, support and slack for any unachieved undertaking, (no one would expect anything of us from a 'sickbed'.) Since this kind of 'sick compassion' is so often the case, we need to ponder an obvious question. What would happen if we became more loving, forgiving, kind, supportive and understanding to ourselves and to those around us as a general rule? At the very least the normal 'benefits' for being sick would be benign and at the very most, we would see the real 'benefits' of radiant health.

Health benefits

Does all this healing mean that the desires of our heart should go unrequited? Not necessarily. Desires, although often tainted with limiting beliefs are many times revealing a genuine need. Such is the case with the following sick turned 'health' benefits. Like food for the body, these needs nourish the soul or whole of us. And like physical food, these spiritual needs are not optional.

*The need for <u>attention and love</u>

*The need to <u>choose our own life</u>

*The need to be <u>free from artificial standards</u>

*The need to do things that <u>make us happy and excited</u>

*The need for <u>time alone</u>

*The need to <u>face life head on</u>

*The need to have a <u>life and work that is self fulfilling</u>

*The need to be <u>free from stress and burden</u>

*The need to be <u>sympathetic at the expanse not the expense of our own happiness</u>

*The need for <u>self forgiveness</u>

We will need more than just one go around of this self evaluation to realize how tied we are to these 'benefits'.

It will take constant self observation and reflection on each of the desires in this exercise to see how much they sabotage our health at every turn. But awareness, like possession is 9/10ths of the law; the law of healing. With that honest awareness, we will begin to satisfy these needs and desires positively through our minds instead of negatively through our bodies.

The end of the 'B.S.'

After these four revealing exercises, it is hard to fathom that our society still hopes to find the answer to chronic aches and pains in better health care coverage or a cure-all pill. Fortunately, we don't have to wait until society gets their heads together about the mind/body connection; we know the truth about the 'B.S.' Limiting Belief Systems, particularly those of a 'personal' nature are what chronic health problems are made of. As we reveal and heal the personal Belief Systems, the purpose of Part II, the body is automatically freer, more at ease, in other words, healthy.

The prevailing belief has been that each of us has a different body. But anyone trained in the molecular structure of the human physiology will tell us that everybody's *body* is made up of the same exact physical matter; electrons. Since that is true, it doesn't take a nuclear physicist to realize that there must be something else, something other than the physical body responsible for one person's headaches and another person's hay fever. That something is obviously our beliefs; the only part of us that is truly different in each person. Through the four 'personal' exercises, we have seen that it is our mind, not our body, that 'catches' dis-ease. It is our responsibility, if we want to live truly well, to catch the sick benefits in the mind before they wreak havoc. To believe that traditional health care practices can really heal us without understanding our belief systems, is the 'B.S' that got us into this chronically sick state in the first place.

Getting to and through our own 'B.S.' is not for the faint hearted.
It takes a unique and dedicated person to work at this kind of healing. Anyone who has remained open to hearing all that has been
discussed thus far should be commended. Let's face it, the principles we have discussed are not about changing hairstyles. These
principles questioned and cracked the very foundation, (though it
was shaky to begin with), of our health system; a system that up until a few years ago, any questioning of it was regarded as a sacrilege. It takes courage to even begin such a nontraditional path.
But once the healing is realized, a healing that is felt on every dimension of our being, society's beliefs on health have no bearing on
our soul. We know the truth and the truth sets us free at last from
the good or bad opinion of others.

As we conclude Part II, *Getting beyond our personal 'B.S.'*, we begin to see what holistic or 'wholistic' health *really* means. This
'whole' new path leads us not toward an outside cure of our *body*
but rather toward an inside healing of our *being*; physically, mentally and spiritually. The last two parts of this book, *Breaking the
Bonds with our chronic ills* including the *Transition* (Part III), and
True Self Healing, (Part IV), get to the heart of this 'whole being'
ideal.

Part III:
Breaking the Bonds with our chronic dis-ease

The term 'bonding' has become a symbol of the new generation of thinkers. We all know the indisputable value of parent and baby 'bonding.' Many marriages, old and new have been elevated to grander heights as husband and wife learn to truly bond. And who can deny 'male bonding' from beating the drums and chanting to feeling the camaraderie at football games, or just over lunch. In the spiritual sense, one that is not normally considered, the intimate bonding with our inner self can be the most fulfilling bond of all.

Once a true bond has been created, knowingly or unknowingly, the connection is so powerful that unless consciously broken, it can last a lifetime. In the case of parent and child, husband and wife, friend and friend, us and our innermost self, this bonding can bring happiness, success and peace. But as with anything else, there are two sides to every coin. Just like we can positively think about the most negative of ideas, (fear, failure, problems), we can positively create the most negative of bonds. Health is no exception to this rule.

The cause of chronic aches, pains and ills has always been an enigma and until recently the search has been on external causes. Only because of much frustration and very few solutions has the search turned inward. The 'bonding' process, well accepted in all other areas of life, is now getting its due respect with health.

Breaking the bonds with our chronic dis-eases while building new bonds with radiant health, is the purpose and the promise of Part III. Realizing the magnitude of the healing power within us, isn't it time we use it to break the bond and the 'bondage' with illness?

Writing a whole book with only half the story

Originally this book was to begin and end with the Personal 'B.S.' We believed that the General 'B.S.', the Metaphors, the Sick and Tireds and the Sick Benefits were more than enough to raise a person's health awareness to a whole new level. That premise was about ten years and five book drafts ago. For some reason, **Health beyond** *Belief* just would not come together back then; probably because much of health's limiting belief systems were still beyond *us*. It would take banging our heads against many brick walls before we could see that we had gotten ahead of ourselves. Before a person could believe, let alone heal their personal 'B.S.', (especially if they were to understand ideas like 'sick benefits'), they had to be well prepared. The problems with health today, we later realized, were not just of a *personal* nature, but of a *universal* nature first and foremost. If a person still held to the beliefs that health was the exception to the rules of creative control and goal achievements, that it was basically the responsibility of the Health Care System, that not being sick was the top echelon of health, and that health was primarily a physical issue, (leaving us waiting and waiting for the miracle 'cure' to be invented or discovered), then any real change would be impossible. Ideas like the metaphors of life to health would be quite humorous for entertainment purposes but would be laughed at as a real source of healing. No, the universal, societal 'B.S.' would have to be revealed and healed and a new foundation built for the personal 'B.S.' to be taken seriously.

The missing 'peace'

So that was it; we had completed the search for the 'B.S.' or so we thought. The old foundation of fear, limitation, misguided responsibility and false concepts of healing - the universal health 'B.S.' - was beginning to crumble. With a reconstructed foundation of faith, unlimitedness, right responsibility and the real source of healing - the universal health truths - the more subtle 'B.S.' could be healed. We could successfully break the personal beliefs from the general ("I get a cold 2-3 times a year") to the most specific, (pain as an atonement for sins). Any personal health limitations said or thought on a regular basis like, "Life is such a headache", or "I'm so sick and tired of this happening in my life," were now 'ripe for the picking'. With our more developed inner vision, we could *pick out* the 'B.S.' at the most subtle of levels. Without such a study of beliefs as was done in Part I and II, how many of us could see our own 'B.S.'; particularly when the underlying fact was that we frequently *benefited* from being sick? Seeing a benefit like *escaping from burdensome responsibilities* with headaches or a serious ill, takes a well developed sense of 'in' sight.

Even with all the revealing and healing of both the universal and our most personal 'B.S.', there was still a missing 'peace'. People with whom we worked, ourselves no exception, couldn't seem to let go of their own specific health problem. Whether it was sinus problems or sciatica, chronic eczema or chronic exhaustion, there was one common thread in all the individualized ills. Each person clung to their chronic complaint like it was their own 'flesh and blood'; which is exactly what it became.

The inner bond to our outer condition

We can argue for a lifetime that "our" condition is the exception to the rule of mind/body oneness; that just because it is *with* us doesn't mean it was created *within* us. We can probably get many people to agree with us, "How unfortunate that you keep getting those headaches," some might say. "Isn't there anything the doctor can do for your sinus attacks?" others may comment. Or the old "There is nothing you can do for that hay fever when the pollen count is up." But the basis of a truth or a universal principle is that if it is true for one condition, it is true for *all*. (Thank God, we can trust that it be so.) Such is the case with the 'bond issue'. For every chronic condition, there is an inner bond to soundly support it.

When we do personal consulting with our clients, particularly in the effort to change a chronic condition, we listen very carefully for the 'bond' that connects each person with their problem. Working with hundreds of people allowed us the experience to prove that for every problem that "just won't go away," there is a bond behind it. We could consult with a hundred different people on a hundred different issues and whoever was willing to reveal and heal the inner bond would see success with their outer condition. So often we are asked how we can help one person lose weight, another raise their self worth, and still another relieve their physical pain. Do we have that much knowledge on so many different issues? The truth is we don't but then again we don't have to.

When working with principle, detailed knowledge is unnecessary. We know little about the intricacies of losing weight, self worth and the scores of aches and pains that face us. What we do have is knowledge and experience on the principle of mind over matter and the power of belief systems; the bond concept is just a subtler form of both. In other words, the principle that 'bonds' a person to their problem, whatever it may be, is the most important knowledge that we need to know. "All other information is just details." As long as we listen closely and help ourselves and our clients identify what is going on within, a bond is always found. We need not become experts on each individual subject, (although some basic knowledge is necessary.) Our job, we found out along the way, is to 'hear' the bond and work together to create a stronger bond with their desired goal. Sounds simple; it is. But *easy*, that's a whole other story

Pet peeves

"You did *what*?" Doreen's fiancee was rather upset at her recent addition to their soon to be shared home. It was a harmless little kitten in Doreen's eyes but Allen saw it as a much bigger threat. Whether it was because of his belief that a pet should be a mutual decision (getting a pet without his consent is definitely one of

Allen's pet peeves), or the fact that a cat could threaten his health, this little addition almost ended their relationship.

Since Allen was a child he suffered from major allergy attacks. Whether it started as a label stamped in his mind by a well meaning doctor or other 'allergens' in his home life, bottomline, he was bonded to them like glue. (Interestingly, his twin brother was 'allergic' to the same things with the same major intensity.)

The worst of the 'allergies', so said the authorities was cat hair. Doreen, not realizing the fear of an allergy sufferer, as allergies are not one of her bonds, didn't think the kitten would be a major problem. Allen considered the new kitten not only a threat to his sinuses, but a slap in the face. However, it was his fear of his 'allergy to cats' that kept him from bonding with any cat at all. While Allen was still angry about the betrayal part of this scenario, it was not a good time for Doreen to suggest that his allergies may be 'B.S.' This was 1985, Doreen was only beginning to explore this 'mind/body' issue herself. Ironically, it was the end result of this happening that made believers out of both of them.

When Doreen realized the *insult* that she had added to Allen's *injury,* (she had not acknowledged his feelings or the severity of his allergies), she apologized. After Allen realized that he had overreacted, they made up and decided to keep the kitten. As they were making up, the kitten crawled on top of Allen's chest, nestled in his neck and went to sleep. Fearing an attack, (anger and allergy), Doreen went to grab the little instigator when Allen said, "No, leave her." That was it, instant bond! Over ten years later, Allen and *his* kitten (now cat) are the best of pals. Markey (a mutual agreement on the name), often gets more kisses from Allen than Doreen does. All without a sneeze or a wheeze from day one of the original 'bonding' experience. Allen's twin also has two cats now and like Allen, a real 'hands on' approach to them.

Where did the 'allergies' go; allergies that were such a major part of both brother's lives for twenty years? Did they 'coincidentally' disappear when the fear and the anger disappeared? Did Allen's *bond* with his cat automatically cancel the *bond* with his allergies? Perhaps he found that there could be more 'benefits' from having a cat than having an allergy. To this day, no one really knows the 'thought' that broke the camel's back; as it wasn't a conscious choice; everything happened so quickly. What mattered most was that Allen decided to keep the cat and get rid of the allergies; it certainly could have been the other way around. Allen has since repeated this story with much humility to several people whose 'dander' gets riled at the thought of cat dander.

The truth and 'B.S.' of allergies could make for one 'health' of a debate. Is it the *thing*, (cat hair, pollen, cigarette smoke), that makes us sneeze or the *thought*? Clinically speaking, it could be proven that the allergen makes us aller*gic*. Fortunately for us, we are *spiritual* not *clinical* beings. We are entitled to 'dominion over' the plants and animals of the world, if we choose to accept that right. At one point or another, we all have accepted that right. Consciously or subconsciously we all have *broken the bond* with negative habits, conditions, ills or people in our life. Science could prove that this *thing* causes this *effect*; but we can all prove otherwise. Life experience is always more reliable than laboratory experiments.

A 'sick bond'

For many reasons, (some of which have been well explained already), a great percentage of people take great pains to protect their chronic ills. From defending their innocence in having it, ("I don't know why this keeps happening!"), to making sure everyone who they know knows about their 'condition'. ("How's your sciatica?"), we can rehash the 'B.S.' in Part I and II of this book, like believing that a little pain is about as good as it gets or any one of the sick benefits already discussed. Reviewing always helps; as we grow in consciousness we can better see the subtleties. If, however, we have exhausted the beliefs and still seem to cling to a chronic problem, even 'protect' it to some degree, there is one level of 'B.S.' we have yet to uncover. Somewhere, sometime and for some reason, we have *bonded* with our chronic condition; if we hadn't it wouldn't be chronic. If something keeps coming back to us, we are connected to it in a strong way. And health problems are no exception to this rule.

This 'sick bond' concept is another one of those 'never discussed' at family gatherings or small dinner party topics. To insinuate to a traditional health thinker that they may be *bonded* with their bursitis, headache or sore feet may just 'break the bond' that *we* have with this person. This bond concept is like calculus; it takes intense study of the basics and a good comprehension of the principle behind it all, before more advanced knowledge can be understood and then accepted. It is for that reason that this powerful bond concept is saved for Part III of this book and the second half of our workshops.

Dare to ask

Perhaps it goes back to our rebellious natures or maybe we believe a medical degree is not necessary to question the whys and wherefores of health. For years we questioned and were determined to find out why one person suffered from neck pain while another has never experienced such a sensation. Where did one family member pick up chronic headaches while a sister cannot seem to get rid of her stomach disorder? Physically, it could most likely be shown where in the body the degeneration is located; but sometimes it cannot be found. Our question, if we dare ask it, is *why* it is there in the first place and *why* with treatment after treatment does it keep coming back? As they say in numerous advertisements, "Ask your doctor." Well, we say the same thing. Ask your doctor why a condition becomes chronic or how it got there in the first place. If the answer does not include some reference to the mind, belief systems or inner dis-ease, get a second opinion.

Of human bondage

For almost every person there exists a chronic condition and for every chronic condition there exists a bond. To say that this bond is the sole reason for the condition depends on whether upon breaking the bond the condition totally disappears. *Some conditions are that easy to eliminate.* But to say that there is absolutely no connection between the strong identification that we have with our particular problem and the fact that it has been with us for years, makes true healing impossible; and the chronic condition remains *chronic.*

If we defend our innocence in our chronic condition or work to prove that this condition is 'really physical', we keep our ego intact, but forfeit any sort of healing. If, on the other hand, we remain open to the possibility that we are unknowingly blocking our own unlimitedness, (even if we can't see the block), our ego may get bruised in the process but our body can truly heal. We do not need to see all the 'B.S.' in our minds nor have 100% faith in the healing power within us for it to work. A shift in thinking can begin a healthy shift in our body. This healing power needs only to be pointed in the right direction; it knows the way from there.

There are many reasons that our body *initially* becomes *dis-eased,* from migraines to missing ease and exuberance, (our natural state), any one of the eight 'B.S.' discussed in Part I and II could be the culprit. Why our body *remains* in this less than radiant state and why the condition becomes chronic (keeps coming back), is a 'bond' issue. A bond is defined as *something that binds, fastens or confines; something that ties a person to a certain line of behavior; the attraction between atoms in a molecule.* In other words, an attractive force within the atoms of a substance binds, fastens or confines it to another substance. Unless one is familiar with physics or Einstein's discovery that everything in the universe, physical, mental and spiritual is nothing but energy, ("Energy Is"), than it would seem to the naked mind that every substance is made up of something different. From this thinking, we would see the air as one substance and the ground as another. Under that premise, the truth that mental thoughts, beliefs and images are powerful forms of energy would never seem logical. It has been well proved however, that whether we are talking about a mental image or a physical illness, there is an attractive force within the atoms that binds and bonds the substances together. More to the purpose, being unfamiliar with the law of energy would cause us to look at the human body as a multitude of different substances; the heart as one substance, the skin as another and the immune system, (where is the immune system, anyway?), as yet another.

What is that attractive force that results in such a bond? For human beings the connecting force that binds a person to a particular condition or circumstance is their degree of consciousness; their thoughts, beliefs and mental images. This brings us right back to the principles of "as a man thinketh in his heart so is he," and "what you can conceive and believe you can achieve." No matter how we slice it, the outer circumstances of a person's life always comes down to their inner state of being. This bond concept poses not a new principle but a deeper connection with the old one. The bond concept explains the mind/body truth as it relates not just to conditions but the *chronic* conditions. Through an attractive force within the atoms of a substance, (and all substances from money to migraines are made of atoms), we attract conditions to our life; positive and negative. The more we mentally bond with a condition (believe that it is inseparable from us or our life), the more we will see it cling to us for dear life, which it has essentially become. The premise of bonding is that it is no respector of conditions. It will fasten us as easily and effortlessly to chronic sciatica as it will to chronic success. Somewhere, we chose the bonds that we have today (most unknowingly), and until broken, these bonds like riding a bicycle, will continue for life.

Yours, mine and ours

Think of the adults with whom we spend a fair amount of time. Is there even one person who honestly does not have some chronic ache, pain or health condition? Have you heard them use the word *my* when describing their particular condition? Even more revealing, how many of these people have chewed our ear off at one time describing in explicit detail all about their condition, how bad it is and what their doctor said about it. (Interestingly, this phenomena does not happen with children; children generally do not suffer with chronic pain.) The point is not to analyze all the chronic complainers in our life, (we may be one), but rather to see how vast is the problem of bonding with chronic health problems. It is rare to find a person who does not have some chronic complaint and even rarer to find one with energy, ease and exuberance. Chronic health problems may have become the norm not because they are a normal part of our *being*, but because they are a normal part of our *bonding*. Radiant health or at least far less pain and ills could be just as normal a part of our being if *those* conditions become the object of our bonding.

It is also quite interesting that not only does everyone have a chronic health bond but there are about as many bonds as there are people. Many people have more than one bond and when one disappears, another soon takes its place. ("I used to have sinus problems, now my gall stones are causing me problems!) Why the problem hits a particular area of our body is another story (for more insight into this question, reread Part II.) Part III is to find out why it keeps coming back.

Bonding. . . it's always something

For Doreen the battle raged on the dis-ease side for years. From the time she was a child, 'swollen glands' had become the direction of her ills. Whenever Doreen was 'sick', her glands would come to the surface, literally. Her parents unknowingly bonded right along with her; they *knew* her glands would be a problem several times a year. By Junior year in college, Doreen had had it with her glands. Antibiotics were not even killing the pain, never mind the problem and no other method was suggested. After about two weeks of horrendous pain, (she couldn't *swallow*; not one of the dozen medical professionals that she visited ever asked her if there were something in her life that was hard to swallow), she broke the bond. One sleepless night while trying to ease the pain with hot tea and oreos (the oreos worked better than the tea!), Doreen remembers saying to herself, "That's it - no more throat pain! From that day on there was no more throat pain. Whatever broke the bond, shock, impact or just sick and tired enough to refuse to live with it anymore, it was gone; too bad her bond with *pain in general* was still as solid as ever.

It took several years to create another bond but this one was a doozy. Instead of the periodic bouts with swollen glands, this new bond was a daily event. Six out of seven days a week, Doreen faced each morning with a splitting headache. Some days it would almost dysfunction her, other days she would pain her way through the day. Why she suffered so much and why it hit her head is not totally clear. Perhaps the fact that she was a newlywed of two months when the headaches started, a newlywed whose husband worked day and night and was considering law school. Along with that formula for 'wedded bliss', Pat and Doreen had just signed a lease for their first office. All they had to do now was get some clients so they could pay the rent! Any surprise that these 'major changes turned into major headaches for Doreen.

Whatever the reason for the initial connection with headaches, the bond was clear as day. Doreen had all the classic symptoms of a bond. She referred to her condition as "*my headaches.*" She kept them a secret from everyone; neither her partner nor her husband knew that she was in pain. (Describing our condition in detail to everyone who will listen or using every ounce of energy to hide it from the world are two sides of the same sick coin.) Doreen also *expected*, although unconsciously, that everyday would begin and end in pain, in fact she was surprised when the pain subsided. Thoughts like, "There it is again. . . it's back, I just knew it would be bad today," were as normal as the headaches. What really cemented the bond was the imagination factor. In no way could Doreen imagine life *without* this pain.

Over the next five years the headaches would come and go; some weeks everyday, others only three or four days. The bond was still going strong. It wasn't until Doreen was in the middle of creating the health workshops at Herman's that it all came together; the 'B.S.' that she and almost everyone else that she knew was not just a *belief system*, it was a *bond system*. The solution wasn't just about changing the belief systems; those discussed in Part I and II had already been presented in the workshops at Herman's. The beliefs had been reckoned with, now the bond had to be broken.

Through a revealing and unique series of exercises to follow, the bonds with chronic pain were well on their way to being broken.

Exercising our right to 'tax free bonds'

We don't have to suffer; suffering is a choice, a belief, not a fate or a truth. We no longer need to live with the bonds that tax our life. Living 'tax free', bonding with radiant health or at least a little more ease and a lot less pain is as much a choice as has been chronic pain. Headaches, backaches, stomach problems, muscle pain, allergies, fatigue and all the other chronic dis-eases, clinical research aside, may just fade away once the bond is *revealed*, then *healed*. That is the purpose behind this next exercise. This exercise will prove more revealing, more insightful into our problem than any physical test. If we are open, honest and really question ourselves, this can be the beginning of the end of our chronic complaints. The key is to talk about where we are *now*, positive or negative, instead of where we think we *should* be. Change is made from the present, our present thoughts, feelings and circumstances. Once we are clear with where we are, (these exercises will help us do that), then and only then can we create where we want to be.

Exercise: <u>Revealing the Bonds</u>

1) Explain in detail the condition or problem in the body that we would love to live without. Describe how it affects our body, how it feels, where it is located, when did it first occur? Include any memory or emotional upset or significant life change at the onset of the condition. _____

_____

_____

_____

2) What is the medical term or label for this condition?

_____

3) If you preface this condition with the word "My," write it here: *"My* _____*."*

4) Describe what spurs this condition on.

_____

_____

5) Think back to the thoughts or emotions just before this condition flares up; what are the first signs?

_____

_____

6) Think back to the thoughts or emotions when this condition is in full manifestation. _____

_____

7) Which side do we find ourselves on: a) talking a lot about this condition to anyone who will listen, b) avoiding talking about it at all, wanting to hide it? _____

_____

8) Think deeply on whether this condition is subtly anticipated or expected or checked for to see if it is there.

_____

_____

9) How does this condition or pain interfere with your life? (be specific) _____

_____

_____

_____

10) Which is a stronger, clearer picture at this moment; my life: a) always *with* this condition to some extent, b) *without* this condition in any shape or form ever again? _____

Let's take a look at the answers that were exposed in this last exercise. Are there any surprises or shocks with any of the answers? "Revealing the Bonds" is one of those exercises that gets a big reaction in our workshops. Few people realize how connected they are with their particular ache, pain, ill or general state of exhaustion. The bond concept is just as true with any area of our life from success to self esteem and the exercises in Part III can be used to heal these areas as well. When it comes to health or health problems, contrary to normal 'health' education, breaking this connection is often the only way it will go away.

The bond concept may be new to our health thinking but it makes logical sense. If the exercise revealed how vividly we can describe the problem, use the word "my" and/or know the medical term, talk about or hide it, expect it, can't imagine life without it, and even subtly check for it when it has subsided, is there any question as to why it follows us around like a lost pussycat? There is good news to this bond concept. If it were revealed through the previous exercise that we *are* bonded to our chronic problem, all we need to do is *break the bond.* This is a far easier task than trying to fix the problem; remember we have been trying to fix it all along and it's still with us.

Equal opportunity bonds

Of course it seems that a bond with a serious problem is stronger and more difficult to heal than that of a minor problem. Not so, a bond knows no bounds. How many times have we had an ache, pain or health problem that we never have had before, even one that someone else gets chronically and for us, it is never heard from again? More times than we realize. Unlike the person who gets this problem again and again, we just never developed a bond with it. (Without this awareness, however, we can bond with this new problem as easily as we did with our old one.) This bond concept explains why we find ourselves more quickly getting over a serious problem that we never have had before than a minor pain that we get all the time. It is not the seriousness of the problem that determines the healing, but the seriousness of the connection. Dr. Eric Butterworth, a wholistic clergyman, emphasizes this bonding process in a story he tells of a true wholistic doctor. Upon hearing that his patient had 'come down' with a serious illness, this doctor had some words of healing wisdom. "I am not worried about the symptoms in your *body,* he said, 'we can handle that. But for God's sake, keep the symptoms out of your *mind.* If it gets cemented there, we are doomed." All doctors should be taught to impart such wisdom.

There is no way around it and no exceptions to this rule; if *we* want a change, *we* have to change. On the positive side, as we do change, so does our life. And as we bond to the new desired changes, so our life changes. It is quite an accommodating system.

"My oh my,". . . *the health saga continues*

We are possessive beings. From childhood the word *my* became a major source of our security. First, it was *my* toys, then *my* family. In fact, children cling with such tenacity to "my toys" or "my mommy" that breaking the bond could still be one we wrestle with as adults! In our teens, the bond became *my* boyfriend or *my* girlfriend, followed by *my* car. We see as adults we form even greater attachments with *my* house, *my* spouse, *my* kids and the old reliable, *my* money. We have even managed to take possession on a global level with *my* country and *my* people. As soon as the word *my* prefaces an object or a condition, a powerful bond ensues. Our chronic health problems are no exception to this rule.

If we listen closely to everyday 'health' conversations, at least once the word *my* will preface the condition. "*My sciatica* is acting up again." "I can feel *my allergies* coming on." "*My arthritis* is getting worse." "*My sinuses* are killing me." We have been bonded with our health professional's answers; "*My doctor* told me that this condition could get worse."

It sounds so innocent using the word *my* to describe a condition that it rarely makes an impression on us or the person listening to our condition. After all, it is just a normal way of expressing our health problem. Yes, it has become quite normal to use the word *my* to talk about our condition; it also has become quite normal to *have* to talk about *our* sick' condition in the first place. Are we just as expressive with our health as we are with our health problems? How often do we say or hear, "My energy level is so great!", or "My health is radiant!" Nowhere near as often, in fact, rarely. Now when we think of the mind/body oneness principle, can we see that prefacing our health conditions with the word *my* and talking about them to anyone who will listen, will bond them to us all the more?

In our society we fully accept the bond that occurs between a mother and a child or a bond that occurs between a person and their potential. Depending on how a mother thinks, talks and acts, determines the connection that she will have with her child, beginning in utero. The bond created by a mother can be so strong that when in tune she can sense her child's distress from great physical distances. A person and their potential can be just as powerful. If a person thinks, talks and acts with no limits regarding their goal, they will succeed regardless of the obstacles. Because of the powerful inner beliefs, the mother and her child as well as the person and their goal are bonded to each other. No reasoning person would dispute this truth. Why then do we stop short of accepting this universal bonding principle when it comes to health?

Breaking the bond

The next step after *revealing* the bonds is to *heal* them. This begins by reversing the first exercise, answering the questions with what we *want* to see in our body. Make it logical. If it feels too much like a fantasy or beyond our reach, our mind will reject it. Find a balance between logic and definite improvement. Use short or incomplete sentences to describe this new state. Take a little thinking time before answering each question as we are far more used to thinking in terms of chronic pain than chronic ease. Over the next several pages, we are going to break the bonds with the problems and begin building a bond with more ease, energy and exuberance; at the very least a bond with less pain.

Exercise: <u>Healing the bonds</u>

1) Describe in full detail what you would *love to see and feel* in your body; use as many specifics as possible as though painting a vivid picture: _____
_____
_____
_____

2) Create a *label* for this new health condition: _____
_____

3) Use the word "My" to describe this new label: "*My*_____ "

4) What do you believe can *spur on* this new health condition, what thoughts or what actions: _____
_____
_____

5) Describe how this new health condition and freedom from the chronic pain or ill will *make you feel emotionally:*
_____
_____

6) When someone asks you *how you feel*, how will you answer with this new state of health?
_____
_____

7) Upon *waking up in the morning*, what thoughts will you have about this new health condition to set up the day?

_____

_____

8) How do you see *each area of your life benefiting* from freedom of that chronic pain, ill or fatigue? (Be specific).

_____

_____

9) When this chronic *dis-ease* is long gone from your life, describe how you would feel. You've been granted your *fondest wish for health*. Write it down.

_____

_____

_____

The process of healing versus a 'healing product'

It should be clearer now that healing cannot be found in a pill or a treatment. Healing in the true and permanent sense is not a product, but a *process*. And this process is different for each person. Even if two people have the same symptoms or condition, their needs and reasons for the condition are very different. The exercises and evaluations in this book have been designed to open each one of us up to our personal needs and limits. If each of our fingerprints are different, our healing needs must also be individual and unique.

The healing process is like peeling an onion; there are many layers to get through before we are at the core. Is this just to make it more difficult on us? Hardly. We need to work through our own 'B.S.' to build the strength and confidence in knowing that we can create the life we want. Only through experiencing this process do we develop faith and cooperation with the power within. In other word, by ourselves, inside and out, we are forever changed and enlightened. What pill or treatment can give us that kind of inner growth? Perhaps this universal power has a grand purpose in making us work for and through our own healing. Maybe we are now ready to accept that higher purpose.

The bond and the 'B.S.'

The more automatic and natural the bond, whether it be negative or positive, the more hidden from our view, as the condition seems so 'normal'. Unless a person is engaged in a holistic health or self growth program, when asked if they are bonded, connected or in any way tied to the particular condition that keeps popping up in their life, the answer is a fairly confident "no." The common response is "it just happens to me." There is no area more believed to just happen *to* us instead of being created or bonded *through* us than our health. . . particularly our health problems.

A principle is a principle; if it works for one molecular substance, it works for all. It has already been well proven that a person can be bonded, connected or tied to conditions like success or failure, loving or abusive relationships and a host of other conditions. Then by the principle of energy, the same must be true for health and health problems. Whatever the condition, if it happens on a regular basis, there is something *in* us - being created *through* us - that keeps drawing the condition *to* us. And thank God for that. If we have unknowingly bonded with one condition in our life, then we can knowingly break the bond with that condition. We can also bond with any and all conditions that fulfill our unlimited birthright to abundance, especially health.

Getting the new image

At first glance it may seem like *creating health* takes much more time and effort than *curing health problems.* Aside from eating right and exercising, we have been led to believe that the job of healing our body belongs in someone else's hands. Even though this approach has left our society with far less than radiant health, it still seems too time consuming to take a truly creative role in our health. Yes, it takes time and energy to create health, especially the radiant, fully functional kind. This work is a creative process that goes on for a lifetime if we want a lifetime of true health, but there is another point to keep in mind. Think about how much time and energy has been lost to headaches, backaches, allergies, stiff joints and muscles, colds, flu, fatigue or just feeling blah. What about the time, energy and money lost going to doctors to find relief from what may be an inwardly created bonded condition? So, if we have found ourselves fussing about the exercises and healing work needing to be done, it is quite normal. As we move into the more natural way of living, however, the added time to create greater ease, energy and exuberance pales in comparison to the time and pain inflicted upon us by leaving this process in someone else's hands.

Setting the new image

We know that it is our responsibility to create or 'set the stage' for this new level of health. The last two exercises, "**Revealing the bonds**" and "**Healing the bonds**," prepared us for the last exercise "**Setting the new image**."

Healing is a step by step process starting from where we are at this moment and gradually, logically building to where we want to go. Now that we have revealed what we *don't* want in (**"Revealing the Bonds"**), created what we do want in (**"Healing the Bonds"**), it is time to set the new image with clear, vivid and definite ideas. For this final exercise, use the answers in the previous exercise,

(Healing the bonds) to create in brilliant color what we would like to see and feel in our body everyday. This time, however, there will be no questions to interrupt the flow of our creativity. Use the answers in the last exercise as a guide, separating them into different paragraphs. Be logical as well as unlimited. Use the phrases *I am. . . I have. . . there is. . .* to indicate a present tense situation, as though we already have the health of which we are asking, because in the higher sense, the spiritual sense, we already do.

My New Health Image

_____

_____

_____

_____

_____

_____

_____

_____

_____

_____

_____

_____

_____

_____

DATE: _____

In order to *bond* with this new image, it is suggested to read it each and every day for 30 days. While reading, vividly imagine living and breathing from this new state of health. Take a few minutes to feel this new state of health. Keep this image with you physically as well as mentally.

I just can't imagine

The principle of imagination is used more often than we realize; unfortunately, more often than not it is used to *negate* our goals. It is no coincidence that we frequently use the phrases like "I have no *idea* what it would be like,". . . "I never *thought* of that,". . . "It never *dawned* on me,". . . "I can't *picture* myself,". . . "I just can't *see* this." as the ways we imagine what we can't have or be. If we just listen, our thoughts and words tell the story of our future. We may think that we have *predicted* the future, "I just knew this would never work," but in truth we have *projected* our old beliefs into our new reality. This is as true for health and chronic health problems as it is for money and chronic money problems. The type of physical matter does not really matter; we can project an image of vital health as easily as a vicious headache. We can also project a *can't* image. If we find ourselves thinking and saying (or subtly feeling), "I just can't imagine this condition healing," "I just can't imagine radiant health," "I just can't imagine more ease," or anything else, we will most likely be right. If we must use the negative side of imagination, let it be for something positive. "I can't imagine ever having a problem I can't handle," "I just can't imagine life without radiant health," "I just can't imagine ever feeling old."

Imagine that. . .

The imagination is nothing magical or mystical; it is built upon the law of energy and is a scientifically proven principle. The 'magic,' if you will, comes in when we put it to use. Some people write down their images daily or weekly; others sit quietly every morning or evening and visualize the life that they want. Still others exercise their right to greatness by imagining their life improving while they walk, jog or stretch. There is no perfect procedure or right way. The methods may be different but the end result will always be the same; the image must be absorbed into our being. Eventually, we must feel the new condition as strongly as we have felt the old.

And this feeling comes before the physical manifestation can come into our life.

Is this 'feeling the image' an intense process? Not really. Visualizing or creative imaging is not a *forcing* of an image, but rather a *freeing* of one. The truth is, what we want also wants *us;* the image of a greater life is already within us. It has just been squashed by doubt, unworthiness and belief that it is not possible. Once the doubts, unworthiness and negative beliefs lose their power, our mind is free and clear to create a new image and set the already unlimited image of greatness within us on its natural free path.

Are we having fun yet?

Freeing or creating a new image is an enjoyable and easy process, in fact it can be one of the most inspiring aspects of our life. It can renew our hope and recharge our enthusiasm for life. If, however, we find ourselves fighting or avoiding the process, either we don't yet believe how powerful this imaging principle really is or we are trying too hard. Forcing a picture to appear perfectly in our mind that needs to gradually evolve over time or becoming discouraged because our goal has not yet manifested in our life are the 'warning signs' of trying too hard. It is not us but the Father (power) within that doeth the work, (in the right time and right circumstances.) What *our* job entails is to encourage the mental image with ease, patience and joy and to do the necessary external work in life to support the image. We also keep doing the mental imaging and the external work for as long as we desire the goal to be in our life or until it becomes so automatic that it is who we are. What we *don't* do is try to force the goal to happen too quickly because of fear or impatience; if we do, it will just take twice as long. Authors, scientists, entrepreneurs and philosophers have attested that daydreaming or imaging, allowing the mind and the spirit to inspire and guide them, made the difference between joy-filled success and torture-filled frustration. This book could not have been written without the hours and sometimes days of visualizing what we wanted to see prior to writing each section of the book. This powerful process worked both for us and against us. When we were only seeing the frustration and difficulty of writing, it was like the doors to our creativity shut down, nothing would come out. They were the self-created barriers of fear and impatience, ("who are *we* to write such a book!" as well as "why is it taking so long?" were common extremes in our ego based thinking.) However, when we spent time seeing the book written and at the same time loving the process, it was like the flood gates were open. The words and ideas flowed faster than we could write them down.

Never put off till tomorrow. . .

Dr. Wayne Dyer wrote a book called, "You'll See It When You Believe It." His purpose was to show how the old beliefs of "I'll believe it when I see it," are the main reasons that we never see it. If we wait until the goal is manifested to see it in our mind or believe it in our heart, we will be waiting forever to have it in our life. However, when we do turn this backwards approach inside out, mentally seeing it and spiritually believing it, the odds are in our favor that we will physically receive it, health being no exception to this rule.

There is an old cliché that says "Never put off till tomorrow what you can do today." This cliché does speak the truth about goal success but only half the truth. To speak the whole truth it would need to say "Never put off till tomorrow what you can *be* today." Physically acting on our goals is necessary, but until the being, (the thoughts, images and beliefs), is in line with the goal, all the doing in the world will do little good. Only when our *future goal* becomes our *present state of being* are we in the position to receive it. Spiritually speaking, Jesus said "when ye pray, believe that ye have received it and ye shall have it." He didn't say *hope* that ye will receive it or *wait* to receive it to believe it or just *pray* that ye will receive it. (Nor did Jesus in any way suggest that this principle applies to all goals *except* health.) Jesus was quite emphatic about the present acceptance of our future desires. If we are more scientifically than spiritually minded, however, the energy principle can be substituted for Jesus' proverb. Everything in the universe, from our mental image to our physical health is just different degrees of the same energy. The main characteristic of energy is attraction; energy attracts that with which it is in harmony. Physical manifestations in our life must be in harmony with our mental energy or they could not be attracted to our life. This is a scientific fact of which there are no exceptions. (Concept-Therapy explains this energy principle in great detail.)

Regardless of our current conditions, as our thoughts, beliefs and images become focused on the goal, (the new state), energy can attract the goal (greater health in this case), into our life. This energy principle is the only way a goal can be attracted to or created in our life, health being no exception. We create with our mental energy that which we can see in our physical energy or life.

Once we have mentally energized the new state, (ease, energy and exuberance), we must de-energize the old state of aches, pains, illness, fatigue and suffering. Denying energy to the problem, refusing to focus on or fear the current state is a great step toward becoming the new state. Contrary to popular belief, denying the *energy* does not mean that we are denying the *problem*. We are not *deluding* ourselves that the problem exists, but rather *diluting* the energy to the problem. But let's not kid ourselves, believing that we have received that which we can barely imagine and denying energy to that which may be killing us will take much inner work. Only if we really believe that the goal is worth it will we follow through on the necessary work. Until that time, we will find excuses to give up all along the way.

The balance between hanging on and letting go

This process of visualization or mental imaging does not require perfect detail as one might anxiously assume. It does require that we see ourselves in the position of receiving that which we desire, even if all the details of that desire are not totally clear. Actually, we can never really know all the details or aspects of our goals; they grow and develop all along the way. The writing of this book was a great example of not being clear on details. There was no way that we could have foreseen or known all the aspects, twists and turns of this book. All we could do was visualize a general picture of what we wanted to see, the confidence that the ideas would somehow come to us, and the enthusiasm that we would love the whole job at hand; the rest was *out* of our hands. We had to hold on to the image while letting go of the fear and impatience. Holding on to what is our responsibility and letting go of what is beyond our control is a constant balancing act.

What we 'want' vs. what we 'asked for'

Does this mean anyone who uses the power of the imagination always gets what they want? Yes and no. We always get what we *ask for*; it just may not be what we want Until a person becomes more 'insightful' (able to see their inner thoughts), it is hard to accept that the manifestation in their life was *asked for*, especially if they are negative. This is why it is so crucial to the health and success of our life that we become insightful, observing and feeling our own thoughts, beliefs and expectations. It is the only way to be empowered vs. overpowered by our imagination.

There are many factors that go into play as we watch the manifestations in our health and overall life. Some we may be able to control and some are there to teach us. Our body and our life present an opportunity to create but also to learn. Sometimes what we really want or more accurately what we really *need* overrides that which we *think* we want or need. For example, we may be frustrated that we keep getting headaches and really 'want' to be rid of them, but they continue to present themselves in our life because we 'need' to see what is really causing them so we can let go of the dis-easing thoughts that keep creating them. We must stay open to all signs of guidance, inside and out. Does this mean we just sit around and wait for the 'spirit to move us?' Hardly. Life is a dynamic, learning, changing and moving experience, one in which we need to balance silent inspiration with fervent dedication; as we are guided, we move. And in the process, life happens; sometimes as we planned but always as we needed.

Making the Transition

By this point in the book, it should be somewhat clear that there is a method to our madness. The purpose in Part I was to get beyond society's well laid 'B.S.' about health, leaving us with a more principled foundation from which to work. Part II then led us beyond our personal 'B.S.' responsible for our aches, pains and lack of radiance. The real healing began in Part III. It was explained why our individual problems have become chronic and how to break these chronic bonds. Part III also included suggestions on how to create new bonds that are free of pain and filled with more energy and exuberance.

Now we have hit a transition, both in the healing process and in this book. Enough has been said about *what* we have to do and even *how* we can do it. All that is left now is to just *do it.* Dreaming is the first step, but *doing* our dreams makes them our reality. So, how come so many of our dreams don't come true? The first reason is that we don't do what we planned to do. But what if we *do* all the necessary steps and for some unknown reason we still see no change? "I did all the right things, I broke the bond, made the right images and I still have the same pain." It is at this point that many of us conclude that this mind over matter stuff doesn't work or that our mind just isn't strong enough. We then return to our old way of thinking and give up ever having a healthy pain free body. The sad thing is that we give up too soon.

The missing 'peace' in goal success

If the teaching of belief systems and mental imaging is rare with regard to goal success, especially with health goals, the teaching of the *transition* is practically unheard of. Ironically, it is the transition phase of every life change, health no exception, that ultimately decides whether we 'go home with the goal' or walk away frustrated and defeated. Misunderstanding this transition phase, (a common occurrence as it is rarely ever taught), is the reason that fear, frustration and ultimate failure have become the normal companions of change. Although not generally accepted as such, change should be a calm, enjoyable, successful experience; when we understand the phase called transition, that is.

If change has become a frightening, shunned experience and our goals a neverending cycle of *going for* instead of *getting to*, it is our approach, not our ability that is to blame. We are endowed with the ability to imagine what we want and then attract what we have imagined. Once we better understand what happens during the transition from where we are to where we want to be, change becomes more natural and goal success more normal.

There is one rule, however, that must be followed in any change. We must have *faith in the vision* during the erratic phase of the transition. How, when and where a change will occur or a goal will be achieved is uncertain; the twists and turns can make our head spin. Some changes and achievements come easily and quickly; others can test our resolve to the utmost and take what seems like an eternity. Other changes may go through an upward climb toward their ultimate, while with some, conditions may seem to get worse, even look impossible before success happens. It is during all these ups and especially downs that having faith in our ultimate vision, seeing what we want versus what appears to be at the time, that carries us safely through a sometimes rocky road. It will often take repeated reinforcement of this vision, (what we want no less than our right and resources to attain it), in order for our vision to win out over the temporary happenings of transition.

It will seem that we are being tested, like forces beyond our control are testing to see if we have the patience as well as the faith to make it. Why else would a simple goal have to go through so many crazy stages? And our mind will do its strongest evaluating, calculating and generating the conclusion that "we just don't have what it takes." But when we look at the transition from a microscopic, fertilized ovum to a fully matured baby, we would never think that some force is testing the mother. And yet, if that part of the process of creating a child was frozen during the first few weeks of conception, a human baby is the last thing one would expect to be born. Before taking on any characteristics resembling a human being, a fetus must pass through stages resembling a fish, a frog, even a rabbit. We consider these awkward looking stages of development totally normal. Remember, a principle is a principle, no matter what we are relating to, transition being no exception. As our goal or change evolves, it will take on characteristics resembling 'going in circles' if not 'total failure.' Who can say that the transition of our goal doesn't need to resemble a 'fish' for awhile? This is why the one rule, *faith in the vision* is so paramount, especially knowing the awkward, sometimes fear inspiring, hope robbing stages that may occur. This faith, coupled with a vivid, continually refined mental picture can be our port in a rocky sea when it seems like our goal will never pass the 'fish' stage. . . but have hope, it will.

Master 'in between'

The word transition means passage from one stage or position to another; not lasting or eternal, an intermediate place. This is an important point to keep in mind when it seems that "things just aren't working." It can be an awkward, fuzzy period where it feels like we are hanging upside down in a cocoon with no trace of butterfly wings anywhere. Before any goal can really 'fly', it must go through an in between stage, a stage that is no longer 'what was' but not yet 'what will be.' As we master this in between stage, (the transition), and become comfortable hanging upside down for awhile, risk and change no longer scare us. And once risk and fear have died out, what won't we go for?

Transitions have become a challenge to master in all areas of life. As much as we think that we are prepared for graduating school, changing jobs, getting married, getting divorced, having a child or retiring, at this point the human species does not adapt easily to change, whether it is a desired change or an expected one. This difficulty in adapting or resisting change is directly or indirectly responsible for stress that never ends and goals that frequently fall by the wayside. School, job, marriage, children, retirement are the normal, well known 'rites of passage' in life, but health is a new area to be included in this perpetual problem of resisting change. Whoever thought that we would resist a change in health, particularly a *positive* change? Too few unfortunately. This is just another example of society viewing health as the exception to the rules that apply to all other goals. The transition between dysfunctional to functional health or functional to fully functional health even though a most wonderful change, can be a challenging one. And although it is not a normal course of study in health education, understanding the transition phase in general and how it applies to health specifically can be a Godsend.

We can never control or predict when or where our goals, greater health in this case, will happen; this is up to a power greater than we and far more qualified. We cannot control change but we can make the transition phase easier, more comfortable and more successful.

Clues vs. Warnings

Change and the transition between the old state and where we want to be was meant to be a natural, free flowing experience; this must be true since change is a constant, never ending process of life. The reason that change and even attaining our most desired and deserved goal have become such a problem is back to our 'B.S.' We can safely say that all problems in life are directly or indirectly related to our 'B.S.' During the transition from the old state to the new, we often misinterpret the signs. We perceive what is a natural process on the transitional path (the fish stage), as us being way off track. The twists and turns that naturally occur during transition rattle our beliefs, (as they should), and instead of working to heal the 'B.S.', we believe it instead. Since we have never been taught otherwise, when what we see during the transition inspires beliefs of fear of failure or unworthiness, we just naturally believe our beliefs and normally begin to give up. If instead of believing our beliefs, especially those that get naturally shaken during any change, if we heal them, our goals are far more likely to be attained and our life draining 'B.S.' begins to lose its power

Getting comfortable being uncomfortable

Since we know change and transition were meant to be a free flowing experience, let's not confuse free flowing with free from discomfort. If there is one thing that can always be predicted with this most unpredictable experience called change, it is that our comfort level will be shaken. Mentally, physically or both, we will experience anything from mild ripples of energy to major rumblings of discomfort. In order for change to come *to* us, a change will need to come *from* us. Whether we call it a change in consciousness, or a new state of being, *we* must be different before anything different can happen. And the inner difference has been described as a period of discomfort, uneasiness, stress, anxiety, even pain. Yes, change and the transition period before the change is complete can be uncomfortable at certain times. Uncomfortable however, need not be unpleasant. As we make peace with the sometimes erratic changes of change, become *comfortable* being *uncomfortable*, we along with the energy of the universe can flow freely as both were meant to.

The path towards successful transition begins with viewing the natural events that occur as *clues*; clues that we are heading for change instead of *warnings* that we are headed for disaster. Although there may be additional ones that occur for us individually, the following are the 'universal clues', those that most normally occur during transition. They are clues that the transition is working but they are also clues that our beliefs, the life draining ones are also working. While we view these clues as positive landmarks on the road to transition, it would be wise to heed the potholes. The beliefs that get stimulated can be overridden, which will help us succeed with our goal, but they can also be healed once and for all which will help us succeed with our life. Either way we win.

Clue # 1: The hold of the old

Pat's dad had a rough time with the transition called retirement. An extremely successful businessman who achieved financial wealth by the traditional 'work 14 hours a day' model of the 1950's and 1960's', he was a tough boss and perfectionist. To Al, work was purposeful and joyful, and during those working years, there was room for little else. His work ethic did help hundreds of people to realize their dream of financial success but after thirty years of dedicating much of his life to his people and his business, it was time for Al to move on. His son was well prepared to take over the helm, as he had been trained to do so for many years, but Al wasn't quite ready to let go. He justified for about three years why he shouldn't retire. At the same time ironically, his health started to decline. Feeling pushed out, tossed aside, worth-*less*, (although Al himself had set the date for his retirement years before) were operating below the surface. Refusing to listen to these strong feelings, his body began to shout them loud and clear. Shoulder pain, chest pain and nervous anxiety were some of the missed messages. The 'hold of the old', even with the great benefits of the new was working overtime on Al's whole being. Even when the new state promises to be a glorious experience, better in most cases, it is normal to want to hold on to the old. This is a clue that change is happening, that we are in transition which is where we want to be. If, however, the hold is actually *holding us back*, it is also a clue that we need to heal the belief that letting go and moving on is a dangerous place to be. Making peace with letting go, even letting go of something painful, is a major growth step in our spiritual evolution; it also allows for easier and faster attainment of our goals.

Fortunately for Al, he was also very much involved in studying and teaching Concept-Therapy, the philosophy that had helped him to heal some major ills thirty years prior.

This new role helped him to let go of the old. Over the last two years, beginning to understand what true purpose in life means, Al has been actively working through the transition to the next stage of his life. He now sees more clearly his purpose in this new phase of life. Although retired from his original business, Al's new career, one that he created himself, is helping others attain abundance on *all* levels. For thirty years, Al has helped people become *financially* wealthy; now he helps people become *spiritually* wealthy as well. Through his teaching, counseling and most important by his own example, Al's life, though still actively in transition, is a great example of transitioning through all the ups and downs, to a grander purpose. Al's purpose is contributing each day to helping others raise their own spiritual consciousness. With such a purpose, he can't help but reap the rewards of a more fully functional life, his health being no exception.

Holding on to the old state, mentally or even physically is normal, even expected when the old state has been *good* for us. But what is the rationale behind holding on to the old state when it has been *bad* for us? Unfortunately, the belief of holding on to the old works just as strongly with something that is obviously killing us. The same problem with letting go occurs with pain, abuse, failure and dis-ease, (the exercise on the bond with our health problem proved that.) It is normal to hold on to the old state, even a negative state; it is a clue that we are in transition. But as said before, if the holding on keeps *going on*, it is a clue that healing of this belief is also necessary.

To say that transition from the old state to the new, particularly with retirement, can be trying is true. To say that we can, depending on our beliefs and purpose for the change make the transition an easier one is also true. Doreen's dad viewed retirement in a totally different light than had Al. Much younger than Al was when he retired, Stan couldn't wait for his last day as V.P. of Finance, although he did realize that he would have to 'do something' with his life. Stan was very aware that a new purpose for his being had to be created and he was more than prepared, beliefs and all, for the new role. Weightlifting had always been a hobby and pleasure in his life, now it became his new career. Over ten years later, Stan still spent a good part of his week at the gym. He was far healthier than he had been ten or even twenty years before. One might attribute this greater health to his dedication to the gym. We will go further to say that it was his dedication to enjoying his life that was the real health accelerator. With a belief that retirement meant 'doing what you love' (not ceasing to be useful) and with a purpose for that love, Stan moved through this transition with ease.

Clue # 2: Split in two

"It changes your life," says just about everyone who has had a baby. As soon to become parents, we nod and really believe that we understand their words of wisdom; we certainly have read all the latest baby books, subscribe to Parent's Magazine and have yet to miss one of our Lamaze classes. But no matter how much we read, plan and prepare, living the change called parenthood versus listening to other people's stories can be like night and day.

Pat and her husband Don had talked quite a lot about having a child; being married seven years they were both ready. The birth of Caitlin Rose was an immense joy for both Pat and Don, as the birth of almost every child is. But the change, the transition from just the 'two of them' to the 'three of them' was experienced differently for 'each of them'.

Cait's birth heralded a new era in Pat's life more quickly than it did in Don's. Even though Pat expected to go back to work right after the baby was born, 'business as usual', the ideas in her head changed the second that Cait popped out of her body. Pat's previously all-consuming career quickly took a secondary role, she would soon, however, have to face the not quite thought out transition from full-time career to full-time caregiver. She gave that transition little thought during those first six weeks of motherhood. But when the six weeks were up that she had allotted for 'transition', the door to her feelings of pre and post motherhood feelings flung wide open.

Pat had worked at some type of job since she was 18 years old. For several years prior to Cait's birth, she had her own business and taught monthly Concept-Therapy seminars, never missing one seminar in seven years. (The birth of her daughter was literally held off until the weekend seminar was over; Cait was born less than 24 hours of Pat's last lecture. With all this work mindedness as a large pat of Pat's nature, the battle began between the old and the new, the old work beliefs and the new life of motherhood. Old beliefs that a person's worth is tied to their work, (remember her dad), that a career person should be on the phone or pounding the pavement forty hours a week (staying home spelled laziness), were some of the feelings that surfaced during Cait's two o'clock in the morning feedings. On top of that, with the Herman's account just beginning, Pat felt guilty that she had left Doreen to 'hold down the fort' all alone. (Ironically, Doreen could not have been happier. She had wanted so much to prove her worth in their partnership and to her this would prove to be the perfect opportunity.)

With all of Pat's guilt about not doing a 'real job' (what did she consider taking care of an infant, *child's play?*), there was still a real desire, a genuine love for her new role as mommy. Pat was feeling split in two, a normal feeling during transition. Unlike her dad Al who held tightly to the old state, Pat was split between the old state of careerhood and the new state of motherhood. Feeling split in two is definitely a clue that we are in the process of change, which is where we want to be. But like all other clues, if never passed, this feeling of split in two will split *us* in two; never reaching our goal at the least and dis-ease at the worst. (Being split is another term for stress and stress is another term for dis-ease.) For her sanity and the health of her child, Pat knew that a balance, (mentally as well as physically), between career and motherhood, had to be found. Thanks to Cait and Pat's inner work on this outer dilemma, Pat made a smoother ride of the often torturous transition between full-time job and balancing both career and parenthood. Six years later, (and growing everyday), to some degree Pat has transitioned to a more physically giving and spiritually connected mom/business owner, (this was her vision); a transition that has enriched her life immeasurably.

Meanwhile, Don, Pat's husband had a different twist to his transition. Don was a natural dad and totally at home with his baby daughter. None of the normal daddy fears like holding, changing or playing with a tiny infant were in Don's nature. His career was not greatly affected; it was pretty much 'business as usual'. The transition for Don was more in the realm of *selfhood* than *parenthood*. Always being the 'big man on campus', Don had to transition from sports jock, life of the party, to just playing the game. Don loved being a dad, but like Pat's belief that a mom was not a 'real job', Don unconsciously believed that being a dad was not a real starring role. The old state of being number one and the new state of just being 'one of the crowd' battled unhealed for about two years. Don was split between stardom and fatherdom but was either not aware of the split or not ready to balance the two. Unhealed for that long, it was a matter of time before Don snapped; actually it was his Achilles tendon that snapped.

In March 1993, after a routine basketball game with the guys (and a routine argument with Pat over the yet to be completed transition from sports jock to family man), Don limped in the front door in excruciating pain. After a horrendous night in the emergency room, major leg surgery and three months of therapy, Don decided that making full commitment to this transition from sports star to family man was no longer optional.

Don began to realize that he could still play sports without always having to be MVP unless it was "Most Valuable Parent, which he has won many times over.) It has been several years of transitioning; yes, it often takes years, but everyday there can be great improvement. Of course, the old feelings may still come up, but working from a new image, a new way of living, we create a healthier outlet for our energy, in Don's case, golf.

Slowly but ever so surely, Don keeps working into the new life that supports *his* needs and those of the *whole family* as well. Sure, it was a sacrifice in a way. We often have to sacrifice part of the old state, if not our ego, in order to successfully and healthily move into the new state. Sacrifices, mentally as well as physically made for the good of the whole, often reap little *instant* gratification but in time become life at its best.

Change comes in all shapes and sizes, some are thought about, planned for and greatly desired; these are called goals. Other changes are completely unexpected, unprepared for and not always the most appreciated. Crisis and traumatic experiences fall into this category. In the middle are those sort of thought about, somewhat planned and pretty well desired. For most, Pat and Don no exception, having a baby falls into this category. A baby is one of those changes that is a glorious experience that can at the same time shake the foundation of a family to the core. It is also one of those changes that force us into transition, ready or not. There is no gradual entrance of this kind of change; the new state is upon us before we can say "post partum."

There are many different ways that change enters and ultimately transforms our life. Whether we are forced into change or fortunate to get the change that we asked for, one thing is sure; we need to let go of the old, grab on to the new and survive the stage in between.

Trapeze of transition

Trapeze artists instinctively know how literally to fly through the transition from one swing to another "with the greatest of ease." They let go of the 'old' bar while keeping their eye on and reaching for the 'new' bar. Obviously, if they refused to let go of the 'old' bar or were oblivious to the 'new' bar, the transition would fail and they would fall. Sometimes these artists need to swing back and forth several times before they feel *ready* to let go of the 'old' bar and take on the 'new' one. We may conclude that these artists are good trapezists, and certainly that is true. But looking with a more spiritual eye, it appears that these artists are not just good trapezists, they are really good transitionists, they are in tune with exactly when to *let go* and when to *grab on* and most importantly, to trust the stage in between.

Clue # 3: Overkill

"Don't push", the nurse tells every women in labor just about the time that she feels like a bowling bowl is stuck in her groin. Ironically, they call this the *transition* phase of birth, where the contractions are at their strongest and if it has been a particularly long labor, mom is at her weakest. The baby is in transition between the birthing process and actual birth. Most women at this point would like nothing more than to push out their bundle of joy. As in any transition, however, there is a period of time when our human power must be suspended to allow for a higher power or for the process itself to take over. Pushing at that time, (mentally or physically), out of fear, impatience or just a perpetual need to always *do something* can hinder, prolong and even defeat the end goal. No one can relate better than a woman in labor to the difficulty of having to just wait and do nothing until the time is right, but all transitions, all goals, require this waiting period. If done at the right time, this waiting allows for a pull that puts our greatest human pushing to shame.

The problem with appropriately waiting - another name for 'letting go and letting God' - is that it surely doesn't follow the normal standards of success. If we are not pushing, trying, forcing, even struggling, (so we have been taught), then we will never get ahead or get what we want. Unfortunately, this kind of 'stress' rarely gets us ahead but almost always gets us sick. When our 'blood, sweat and tears' is coming from our fears, when we are afraid that if *we* don't

keep pushing, things will fall apart, then we are blocking the only
power that can put things together.

While it can be hazardous to our health goals, as well as all other
goals, to try forcing things to happen our way and on our time is a
normal transitional impulse. As our life is changing, that fuzzy, 'neither here nor there' period will hit us at one time or another. We
may then begin to doubt ourselves and the likelihood of a successful
change. In order to suppress our fears, we may feel the urge toward overkill; we may want to do anything and everything,
(mentally as well as physically) to hurry things along and avoid our
worst fears. Overkill is another clue of change, that we are in transition between the old state and the new. It is when we are working overtime on overkill, when the pushing, stressing and forcing
don't seem to pass, that we are now blocking the power from doing
its job. Re-centering on the power within as our greatest support
and re-focusing on what has probably become our 'lost vision' will
begin to balance our *going with* with our *letting go.*

So how do we know when to stop pushing and trust the power
within to pull us? There is no universal 'right time'; it is an individual intuitiveness. Back to the trapeze artist, they *just know* when to
let go. Of course, this knowingness comes after much practice *getting to know* the power within. We cannot give an exact formula
for when it is time to stop pushing and allow for a greater pull to
take over but we can make some suggestions. Also, we must stay
clearly aware of and actively work at healing the old limiting beliefs.
For this transition, (our health goal), the limiting beliefs were well
explained in Part I and II. While watching for the 'B.S.' that attempts to block our success, continue to visualize the new health
state in which we want to be. Of course, there are physical action
steps that must be done; a proper nutrition, exercise and recuperation plan must be followed. These physical laws are clearly dem-
onstrated in the Rays of the Dawn book by Dr. Thurman Fleet of
the Concept-Therapy Institute[11]. Beyond these mental and physical

11   Rays of the Dawn, Concept-Therapy Institute, 25550 Boerne Stage Rd, San Antonio,
TX 78255, 1-800-531-5628

actions, a period of *inaction* or trust is required to pull us through. Should we continue to push at the time when letting go is necessary, damage to us or our goal is inevitable. Nothing kills our goal or breaks down the body quite as fast, (from headaches to chronic ills), as pushing too much or too long.

Doreen will never forget the words of wisdom from Dr. Victor Loofboro, a chiropractor and veteran Concept-Therapy teacher of over forty years. During Doreen's battle with headaches, she asked him to help her. He listened to her talk for a few minutes, then felt her head and intuitively knew the 'medicine' that she needed. Dr. Loofboro looked at Doreen and said only seven words: "Let the chips fall where they may." Of course, Doreen would have much preferred a more direct solution; a series of physical exercises, a revolutionary vitamin, even a suggestion to meditate would have been easier to grasp. No, she did not quite understand Dr. Vic's profound words at that moment. Over the weeks, months and years of reflecting on these words, the understanding has come. She now realizes that her constant *pushing* and never allowing the power to *pull* her to her goal not only blocked her goal success, but the mental strain broke down her body. Dr. Loofboro's words to "let the chips fall where they may," is another way of saying to trust that the power knows the road to success, health being no exception. Doreen has since found how a tightness in her neck or a pounding in her head can be healed by ceasing the push and embracing the trust.

Clue # 4: The what ifs

"What if I can't do it?" worried Kathy, a personal client of Doreen's. Kathy had been living with migraines for years before realizing that she had created a bond with them. Doreen had been working with Kathy on breaking these bonds; Kathy had agreed that there was a mental cause and cure for her physical dis-ease. But during the transition from her "morning migraine" as she called it, to waking up free and clear, fear struck. Kathy became afraid that she might not have the ability to break the bond. In other words, she *feared failure.* This was not surprising since fearing failure is a major stumbling block to any change. The prevailing belief is that failure is far more likely than success. (This belongs with the same 'B.S.' that suggests that dis-ease is far more likely than health.)

God knows why we human beings hang on so tightly to the fear of failure, especially when we can tap into a Divine power that *never* fails. This of course goes back to building trust, the only cure for fear. Whatever the root cause, fear of failure is a universal belief system and not understood, is a definite deterrent to transition success. Fear will probably always come up to a certain degree as it is so dyed into the human consciousness. But being sensitive to fear and being sabotaged by it, are worlds apart.

Once again, it is normal to feel uneasy or uncomfortable during transition. And as long as we flow with the uneasiness instead of fearing or fighting it, the so-called negative feelings will lead us to a positive result. It helps to be aware ahead of time, (the purpose of this section on transition) of this uneasiness, dispelling some of the panic. Thinking or saying "What if. . .?" relating to fear of failure is a normal clue that we are in transition. If, however, our 'what ifs' cause us to move away from our goal, physically or mentally, the fear must be faced and healed.

Clue # 5: Castle/Tunnel Syndrome

As we find ourselves definitely on the road of transition, working through the comfort shaking but success indicating clues that clue us in that transition is happening, things may get foggy for a time. By this point, we have probably felt the *hold of the old,* (Clue # 1), where the old pain, problem or fear of illness beckon us to give up our hopes for a healthier being. If we work through this hold and focus strongly on the ease, energy and exuberance of our new health goal, the hold of the old will loosen. Next. we may find our-selves *split in two,* (Clue # 2), not quite 100% focused on the new but certainly not held by the old; we are split between the problem on some days and the power of healing on other days.

Once we make a firmer commitment to the new health goal, letting go of the old state completely, a new sense of urgency may crop up. It is quite normal to become 'over zealous' at the prospect of total commitment. Fearing that things may not work out, there is a tendency toward *overkill*, (Clue # 3), to overcompensate for the subtle panic. Inevitably, this working harder and more anxiously will lead to the twin of overkill, the *what ifs* (Clue # 4.) If overkill is based on fear, it is unlikely that it will speed up the transition; on the contrary, it could slow things down. When the extra 'blood, sweat and *fears*' do little to accelerate success, they tend to accelerate our fears of failure instead. We 'what if' ourselves to insanity until we remember to focus on our goal, not the clues.

Eventually, the "what ifs" and the fear of failure do pass, assuming that we *work through* instead of *falling into* them. Things begin to look up; physically we feel healthier, more energetic, free of pain and mentally we are calmer, more confident and believe in the power of our own healing more than ever. There is now tangible proof that the transition is leading us closer to our goal of more radiant health. But change is change, especially before the change is solidly set and we, no less than the health goal itself, are still in transition. So called 'good' days are bound to be replaced by so called 'bad' days where our whole being couldn't feel worse. The old pain returns, the old fears spring up and we think that we must have been out of our mind to expect such a positive change in our body. We begin to believe that we cannot really create our own health and those around us confirm it. It feels like we have been "building castles in the air", that there is no basis for what we were hoping to accomplish. And now, with our health either deteriorating or at best staying the same, not only do we feel like we are "building castles in the air", but we begin to doubt whether we will ever feel good again, in other words we see "no light at the end of the tunnel." It seems like we have hit a brick wall but in reality what we have hit is another clue of transition.

Clue # 5: Castle/Tunnel Syndrome usually hits deep into the transition. Whether because of slowing down of our healthy mental imaging or the fact that our health needs to go through this cycle before getting better, it is a normal, healthy phase. Having doubts about the 'reality' of such a creative healing process as well as whether we will ever see the 'light' is normal when our goal seems to be stuck in neutral or going in reverse. Obviously, we are in transition; we are trying to make a change or we would never be going through such questioning and anguish. The key, as with all previous clues, is to be *aware* of them, know they will rock our comfort level but never let them ruin our choice for change. Think of these clues as "for illustrative purposes only," illustrating the ups and downs of transition but not the likelihood of it.

Clue # 6: Stress from success

Transitioning can be a bumpy road as the changes we are creating on the outside cannot happen without definite changes on the inside. Doubts, anxieties, frustrations and fears will periodically surface with change, as the fear of failure is often a real concern. But society has become so consumed with the fear of *failure* as a major obstacle to change, it has overlooked a fear with just as much power, the fear of *success*.

Clue # 6: Stress from success addresses the problem that occurs when we finally get what we have so long hoped for. This clue, while normal during the final stages of transition, if not worked through, can kill a goal just as it is about to be born.

"Everytime I get *this close*, I blow it." so many people exclaim in frustration. "I don't know what happens, I had it, then I lost it." "It was here and then it was gone." What may seem like *hard luck*, getting so close to our goal success, but never quite making it or attaining our goal and in the next breath losing it, may just be the fear of success belief.

It took about two weeks of working with Kathy, the now unbonded "morning migraine" person for Doreen to realize the remaining problem. She was experiencing less and less migraines which both Doreen and Kathy saw as a sign that complete healing was not far behind. But just when a week or two would go by pain free, Kathy would "lose it", as she called it and wake up with a splitting headache. Doreen, half joking and half frustrated said to Kathy one day, "Are you afraid of being *well?*"

It took that experience plus working with many people afterwards and observing our own personal 'B.S.' for us to realize that success can rock our comfort level just as much as failure. Being uncomfortable with change does not change just because the change is positive. Although difficult to explain to the average person, positive health changes, moving from chronic pain to more ease and energy can be very uncomfortable. Being bonded with a health problem, ("*my* headaches", "*my* allergies", "*my* stiff neck"), allows us to be mentally comfortable being physically *uncomfortable*. In our unconscious but desperate search for security, our health problem becomes one of those few things in life that we can count on.

Questions need to be posed when we just about have what we want for our body in the palm of our hands. "Can I *handle* having less or even no pain?" "What will I do with my life and my thoughts once the pain, problem or fear of illness are gone?" "Do I feel I can *keep* the greater health when I get it?"

And most important but least considered, "Do I feel that I *deserve* such great health?" ("Have I been 'good enough' to feel so good?") These are not easy questions to think about, never mind have real true answers for them. As we can positively answer them, the last stage of transition makes a turn for the better.

Fearing success - worrying if we can handle and maintain the goal once it is attained, not to mention whether we deserve something so good in the first place - is a normal clue that transition is not only happening, but just about complete. And what was true with the previous five clues is true for this last one; if the clue goes beyond just *clueing us in,* further healing is necessary.

If there is one aspect of this stress from success that needs to be healed with almost everyone, it is our *worthiness.* Where it began may lead us back to prehistoric man, but the current fact is that our society is in great need of work on our worth. Subtle and not easy to accept is our deep rooted belief that we just don't deserve. Further covering up our awareness of this belief but in truth revealing it, is our demanding that life give us what we want. Outwardly demanding is a far cry from inwardly deserving. It has also been proven that any chronic problem in our life has this unworthiness at its base, health problems being no exception to this rule.

Inevitably during the end of the transition between our old state of pain and fear and the new state of freedom from this pain and fear, there comes a time when this unworthiness 'B.S.' kicks in. Just when we start feeling better physically, we may likely begin feeling worse mentally. Attaining what we think we *want* may rattle what we think we really *deserve.*

A host of past guilt, some of which have been discussed in Part II will try to sabotage our newly attained success. Our guilt based mind begins to support our unworthiness thinking. With all the things that we have done in the past and believe that we *shouldn't,* not to mention all that we haven't done that we believe that we *should* have, how could we deserve such a great state of health? And what about all those people around us and on the news, in magazines and on fact based TV movies who are sick, often gravely? Maybe we should be satisfied with our relatively minor problems! We have become comfortable with mediocrity! As hard to believe as it is, a pain free or even pain*less* body may make us quite uncomfortable, especially when deep down we feel undeserving of it. Being clued in on this stress with success, having unworthiness at the core, is a double edged blessing. First, it urges us to heal this unworthiness of greater health, the last fear separating us and transitional success. Second, it urges us to heal our general state of unworthiness, (the king of all 'B.S.'). As we raise our worthiness, *believe* more that we *deserve* more, our life is raised to a whole new level.

In a nutshell

Whether we experience one or all of the six clues of transition will depend on how we handle change in general and health changes specifically. In any case, being aware of the different ways our comfort level may get shaken at times gives us a major advantage; we cannot be blind sided, as happens with so many unsuspecting transitionists, once our eyes have been opened. Let's review the six clues:

Clue # 1: The hold of the old. . . When the old state, the problem or the state that we need to leave has a much stronger hold on us than the new state or goal, *we try to justify why we should "stay where we are."*

Clue # 2: Split in two. . . Being bound to and moving toward neither state, we feel an equal pull from both. We may try to keep both, the old state and the new one, *without commiting to either.*

Clue # 3: Overkill. . . Now committed to the new state out of fear or impatience, we attempt to rush it, force it and/or work and worry ourselves to the bone, trying to *override our subtly rising fears.*

Clue # 4: The what if's. . . More deeply dedicated to the new state or goal, our fears, particularly the fear of failure rise vividly to the forefront of our mind, *a mind now reeling with the 'what ifs'.*

Clue # 5: Castle/Tunnel Syndrome. . . Having experienced definite, positive changes toward our new state or goal, we develop a false sense of security based on outer proof. When the outer proof takes a temporary downward shift, so does our inner faith; we look at our goal as "castles in the air," as if the *light at the end of the tunnel blew a permanent fuse.*

Clue # 6: Stress from Success. . . We are so close yet once again, so far. Just as things begin going our way, we get that gnawing uneasiness that things won't or *shouldn't* last. Used to problems or mediocrity for so long, success and the really good things in life shake up feelings of unworthiness that we *demand a lot, but deep down, believe that we deserve a little.*

There is a delicate balance to be achieved with the six clues of transition; a balance between full awareness of the inner rumblings without being so shaken by them that we allow them to overtake us. Each are normal discomforts that arise during the transitional journey. If the discomforts become dis-easing or dis-abling, however, we are out of transition and into fear; a clue not to panic but to heal the fear and get back on the transitional path.

Healthy transitions

Transitions, (another one of those principles of life that happen *everywhere* but are taught about practically *nowhere*), are a constant in life. Everything in life is either growing toward perfection or degenerating downward; staying the same is not an option. Thank God for that. Since transition is forever operating, we always have the opportunity and the resources to improve our life, health being no exception. In fact, the human body is the epitome of constant change and transition. Contrary to pessimistic belief, the human body is a positive healing waiting to happen. Not a millisecond goes by without a million physical change occurring within each cell of our body. How then can we ever again believe that the *body* stays chronically ill? The body couldn't stay the same if it tried!

Whether we are aware of it or not, we are always in one transition or another. Now as we *consciously* use the principles of transition and become more comfortable with the uncomfortableness of change, what can't we create? At the very least, stress, aches and ills would be far less since these dis-eases are a direct result of re-sisting or fearing change. Life is hard, success is rare and dis-ease the norm not because of *fate* but because we *fight* life's changes. In fact, those people who really enjoy their life and get more of what they desire are those who transition well, who mentally and physi-cally flow with life. Attaining the state of health that we want, free-ing ourselves of chronic pain and radiating with an energy that would make the 'pomp of emperor's ridiculous', are just some of the bonuses that good transitioning brings.

Exercising our right to healthy transitions

Practice makes perfect; transitions are no exceptions to this rule. Unfortunately, change and new opportunities instead of being sought are fought. Risking the obvious, however, we must take and *make* risks a normal part of our life. As we try new things and take a self-created challenge, work through something that had in-timidated us, put ourselves out there when we would rather hide under the covers, life takes a 360 degree turn. Transition is the key to the 'good' life. Moving mentally and physically is the only way to move the energy of the universe. And vowing everyday to making some sort of change in our life is the key to 'good transitioning'.

Part IV

True Self Healing

After decades of being under the domination of the traditional health system and putting almost all of our health needs in someone else's hands, many believe it is time for a total about face. Instead of becoming totally subservient to the system of 'medical healing,' the trend is moving towards 'self healing.' In theory, this concept of self healing seems the most natural and with what has been proven about the healing power within, the most effective. Yet if we make this nontraditional, natural approach just the other polarity of the traditional, medical approach, the results will be about the same; ineffective.

*We cannot escape the truth about healing, regardless of the approach. Healing is a **process**, not a **product**. It cannot be bought, forced or induced externally by some pill or treatment, or internally by our self. Anyone who has been led to believe that self healing means we can just 'think' ourselves well or use a method like nutrition, chiropractic or massage to 'make' ourselves well, is only half right. All natural, nontoxic methods will benefit health to a point. True self healing means that we also work to 'heal the self,' (fears, angers, feelings of inadequacy and guilt) that dis-eased the self and the body in the first place.*

Self healing is the way of the future. To ignore the unlimited healing power within, a power so ready to work for us, would be the greatest barrier to health we could create. It is only when we truly 'heal the self' that we experience fully functional health and a fully functional life.

After searching the world over for the secret to happiness, St. Augustine profoundly stated, "God makes us for his purpose and our hearts are forever restless until they repose in thee." This insight, previously reserved for our systems of religion, is becoming the foundation for our systems of healing.

Nothing causes more outer problems, health being no exception, than our inner unrest. As luck may have it, nothing cures more outer problems, health especially, than our inner repose. For health to reach the glorious heights to which it was intended and to which we are fully entitled, it is time for a profound shift. Whether we call it finding God or connecting with our innermost Self, healing the separation between us and our Divine Self must become a healing principle, not just a religious precept.

True Self Healing, healing the fears, guilt, hurts, resentments and grievances that separate our human self from our Divine Self is our greatest purpose and our greatest privilege. As we heal the holes in our self, the whole of our being and the whole of our life are healed as a matter of course. There are no exceptions or substitutions for this rule.

As we enter this next millennium, we truly are entering a "New Age;" an age that is raising its purpose of life from higher technology to higher self. Elevating this purpose as a society or all by our (Higher) self, we experience a healing of being that brings a healing of body to a whole new level.

Physical health. . . is it all just a front?

There is no question in any sane person's mind that staying well should be a top priority. No one likes being sick, at least not consciously. We feel more alive, can physically do more, have more enthusiasm in our daily work and contribute more to life when we feel good.

Any system that will keep us well, as well as lead us toward radiantly health should be taken very seriously. This book has been devoted to just that end. There is one question, however, that must be answered before completing this health program. Is physical health our *purpose* in life, or is it the *path* to our purpose?

Although we may be immune or oblivious to it, we are besieged each and every day sometimes even badgered with 'health news.' Judging by the huge amount of press on wellness, not to mention the endless warnings about sickness that literally scare the *health* out of us, you would think once we become physically healthy, we are complete. Well, think again. While a worthy goal that should be pursued zealously and actively, the health of our body is not the ultimate purpose of our life. It should, however, be the *path* to our purpose. We may look like a physical entity and our society focuses almost all its attention on our physical, material needs, but our physical being is just a 'front' for a far grander purpose. The true meaning of life is found when we realize that it has never been lost.

If we wish to ever satisfy our needs and longings, health being no exception, there has always been and will always be only one way. As we turn away from the noise of the world, listen unemotionally to the unsettledness in our own mind, a renewed sense of tranquillity will return. Our innermost self not only *has* what we need, it *is* what we need. The answers to our physical desires are found within, but even the greatest of physical treasures pale in comparison with those of the spirit. As we allow for periods of inner solitude to become a priority in life, the fears, guilt and hurts that have too long consumed us, are finally able to heal. Ease and security replace fear; true forgiveness washes away guilt and hurt and as these disappear, a deep sense of love and understanding fills our being.

Being led to believe that health, happiness and peace are found in the technological instead of the spiritual, we fight any inclination toward inner stillness. Instead of 'going with the flow,' the normal tendency is to push outward, overlooking the struggle and pain that come with the territory. It is at this time, when we ignore the unbendable curve toward inner stillness, that we become 'bent out of shape.' From spiritual emptiness to physical dis-ease, our life and our body literally transcribes the suppression of this inner pull; and the harder we try to suppress it, the greater the suffering. Surrendering to the natural bend of the circle of life, the bend back to our Real Self, releases the one true healing power; a power that circles all our healing needs, physically, mentally and spiritually.

For some, this realization that the circle of life always bends us back to our inner self, comes after much suffering and dissatisfaction with life. For others, there is an inborn urge toward spiritual enlightenment that has always had a place in their life. Regardless of what has impelled us toward inner growth, the process can be individually encouraged. As we consciously choose to follow the circle inward, to fill our being with the power of stillness, suffering will no longer be necessary to urge us inward. It will take much less to lead us within and we will find ourselves traveling in much smaller circles.

What 'I.S.' the truth?

Searching for more spirituality in life is not a new concept, nor is it a particularly difficult one. The problem, one that can block the very power that we are born to possess, is *where* we search. Taking an external approach to this intimately internal ideal, looking upward or outward for what can only be found inward has been our greatest downfall. Praying or pleading for divine intervention without elevating our consciousness to a level of divine receptivity is like listening to Mozart with cotton in our ears; the Divine Melody is playing all around us, but we can't hear it.

What we call this Supreme Power of the universe, the spiritual dimension of our life is far less important than *where, when* and *why.* To encourage a healthier approach of *where* we look for this power, in this book we refer to it as the Inner Self. This term leads us to look *inward* for the answers, whereas many spiritual or religious ideals suggest that the power resides outside of and separate from our self. The subtle shift in consciousness, *coming from* a state of unlimited power, versus *looking for* it, makes the difference between a lifetime of searching for the answers and one of finding them. The power, the peace and the healing are and always have been within. We need but take a minute to stop the mad search and allow what 'IS' to become. The Inner Self, 'I.S.', is the *real* us. Like any seed, the Inner Self has all the potential built within, needing nothing more than good tilled soil, (a consciousness that is constantly being healed of dis-eased ideas), and regular nourishment, (feeding ourselves with positive, loving and spiritually uplifting ideas), and quiet time to grow, (periods of inner stillness, gradually becoming a life of outer calmness as well.)

If the *where* of our unlimited power was in need of some healing, the *when* and the *why* will no doubt require the same clearing up to take this ideal from good words to a good *life.* When do we call on this inner power; in times of trouble, if we have a free moment, during religious services? 'I.S.' this Inner Self the very foundation of our life or an 'as needed' or 'emergency' service? 'I.S.' this Inner Self an ideal consistently built upon every day or do we hope and pray that help will magically appear when needed? 'I.S.' the purpose of inner growth to empower our very being or just being there when things get rough? Of course, having the Inner Self on an *always*, instead of a *whenever* basis, is certainly far from the norm for most of us, then again the norm 'I.S.' certainly far from healthy.

Now for the *why* of this ideal. While finishing the last section of this book at one of the local diners, the manager asked us what we were writing about. Always enthusiastic when someone takes an interest in our work, we explained that our objective was to help people connect with their Inner Self. His candid response was quite a commentary on the times. He shook his head and said, "But why?"

The *why* of what we and many others in the self/spiritual growth movement do is actually a vital question. The motive or real reason behind anything a person does, inner self growth no exception, determines the final outcome. As St. Augustine said, "We are made for God's purpose;" all the great philosophers throughout history agree that our central purpose for being is to allow the 'God within', our divine nature, to grow and flow. Anything short of that ends in some level of dis-ease and/or suffering. We are here on this earth plane to enjoy and take part in the physical pleasures it offers, but if the purpose of our life, (the *why* of our self or spiritual growth) is focused on what we can get physically instead of how we can grow spiritually, we may win the battle but lose the war. Spiritual growth, living for the fulfillment of our Inner Self 'I.S.' not an option, no matter how hard we have tried to make it so.

"You can lead a horse to water, but you can't make him drink." In the same light, you can lead a person to truth but you cannot make him think. Spiritual growth, filling up with our innermost self is a conscious, creative choice. Each person must consciously choose to create conditions that serve this end. No one can do it for us, nor can they force, intimidate or even motivate us to get on this path. The light of seeking truth must dawn upon us and within us for it to become the purpose of our being. Sometimes, it takes years of reading, studying, meditating, searching, before we no longer just *say*, "Hark, I hear a (spiritual) cannon," we really hear it!

Although the path of inner growth must be sought for nothing more than the path itself, Jesus seemed to add an extra bonus to the deal. He said to the people of his time, "Seek ye first the spiritual and all else will be added unto you." Fortunately, as far as the truth is concerned, things haven't changed in two thousand years.

Enough is enough. . . or is it?

After the myriad of beliefs presented (more than half of this book has been devoted to the limiting beliefs on health), we could have ended the program. When our students are "up to here" with the neverending 'B.S.' discussed in our workshops, we could stop at that point. After all, enough is enough already. But there are two sides to change, health being no exception. On one side, we must reveal and work to heal the beliefs that keep us from our goal. The illogic, negativity and suppression of human healing potential embodied in today's normal beliefs on health must be seen to be believed. On the other side, one that either is taken for granted or not to be taken seriously, 'I.S.' what lies beyond the 'B.S.', The Inner Self, the unlimited, unconditional and unchanged aspect of every human being, 'I.S.' the only place from which change, healing no exception comes. It is not enough to do the right things; even thinking the right thoughts is only a piece of the peace. Change of any kind comes not from a new *idea* but a new *ideal*. Saying our health image out loud and then doing the plan set forth are the first steps, but when all is said and done, it is our innermost self, the real power within us that makes the difference between a good idea and a healing ideal. The faith, inspiration and strength needed for our goal, no less than our life, comes from opening up to the still, quiet place within. Gradually, following days, months, years of meditation on the power within as well as a conscious daily practice of uniting with this power, we become who we have always been and less the 'B.S.'

'I.S.' the unlimited power limited to a select few?

Grace attended almost all our health and self growth workshops given at her company. She was one of the hundreds of clerks, at the same job for over ten years. Looking at Grace, her demeanor, her overall life, one would have assumed that major life changes were beyond her power. But this woman was a paradox. On one hand, with only a high school diploma, a rather menial job and being over fifty, she appeared 'not to be going places.' On the other hand, for those who really knew her, a quiet but intense power waited patiently to be freed. Even her name spoke of a hidden potential. Grace had humility and a sense of awe about what was missing from, yet possible for, her life. Without this inborn trait, Grace would have been suppressed by a society that believed success was reserved for the young business bound college professional with a degree. Adding to her intuitive genius, Grace showed no trace of resentment for a system that obviously discriminated against people like her.

Grace and so many others quickly took to this principle of the unlimited power within. As the instructors, we certainly promoted the truth that anyone, at any age, level of education, economic standing, state of health, could tap into this power and re-create any aspect of their life. But even we were surprised at the changes that occurred with those who had few, if any of the normal standards of a 'successful person.' For Grace, the releasing of old hurts and current fears, as well as connecting with her Inner Self was amazing. To the shock of her doctors, after years of unsuccessful medical testing, Grace's blood pressure normalized. Personally, she became vitally more confident, outspoken and calmly assertive with her needs. Except for the company policy of a college degree required, Grace now had all the makings of a great office manager. So many more positive changes were made by those students who stuck with working on their Inner Self in the workshops than those who focused on outer changes only.

As Grace smoothed out the wrinkles on the inside, those on the outside miraculously followed suit. For a woman in her fifties, Grace's face had quite a lot of wrinkles. But after a few months of 'facing the world differently', there was an obvious difference on her face. Wrinkles disappeared, taking years off her appearance. Friends and family begged for the 'secret', hoping for the name of a new face cream or a revolutionary vitamin. When Grace explained that the 'secret' was unleashing the hidden potential within, those begging to know quickly begged off. Whether out of sheer disbelief or not wanting to do the work necessary, friends and family dropped the whole idea. Fortunately Grace and so many other students didn't. Those who had truly experienced the Inner Self needed less and less of the outer world's approval.

The point of this story and why it needs to be shared is quite powerful. The Inner Self, the unlimited and unconditional power within is accessible by all. IQ, academic education, college degrees, economic standing, age, sex, job position, marital status, all the outer standards normally equated with a person's potential mean nothing to a person's real potential. The Supreme power of the universe resides within us all and does not require a good resume before allowing entrance. Rather with humility, faith and conscious work on the inner connection, any one at any time can create any change.

'I.S.' today the best time of our life?

There is a tendency to look back over our life with a kind of melancholic nostalgia. "Those were the good old days," is often said as we remember what has been and lament over what is happening or yet to be. Was the past really the best of times or is the thought of the future just encircled with a sense of fear? Are we again limited by a belief system, a belief system that says that the future - *the unknown* - is something to be feared? The less we know about the way life operates, how our whole being interacts and connects with the rest of the universe, (lawfully and logically), the more fear surrounds the unknown. It is not that the unknown is such a fearful uncertain place, or that it doles situations out to us, (particularly difficult ones), with no rhyme or reason. It is just that the rules of life and the laws of our being have yet to be made an educational priority in today's academically focused world.

Fortunately, there 'I.S.' a way to make today the best time of life and thoughts of the future calm and promising. The more centered we are within, the more that we connect with our Inner Self. The more that today is filled with joy, the more tomorrow is faced with freedom. Nothing can match the ease that surrounds our life; past, present and future, than becoming secure with our Inner Self. It is only this deep sense of ease that can heal the dis-ease that seems so unchangeable. Contrary to today's physical belief, the root of our ills are not on a 'cell' level, but a 'self' level; and it is, the 'I.S.' This Self that is our unlimited storehouse of healing - physically, mentally and spiritually - patiently waits to be released.

An external approach to internal growth?

A word of caution; education and evolution are two different things, but both are necessary for growth. We can educate our self with all the spiritual truths ever created, but to evolve, to really change and lift our self to a higher state of being requires a whole other process. The truths, spiritual healing or otherwise, can only become *us* when we become *them*. In this academic world, we can bypass this process by memorizing and verbalizing the required information. But the memorizing and verbalizing process doesn't work in the spiritual world; and believing that it will has led many to disillusionment. The New Age, Self Help, Wholistic, Alternative movement is filled with those who have tried to hypnotize themselves into health and wealth. The majority have the best of intentions but unfortunately the path to health is *not* 'paved with good intentions.'

In desiring a better state of being, we must ask ourselves, "Am I able to receive such a state?" "Is my *head* in line with what I want for my *body*?" Metaphorically, we need to stretch out our hand in order to be pulled upward. God, or the universe can only lift us if we are in a position - mentally as well as physically - to be pulled upward. Peace, abundance, joy and health do not come *to* us as the world will have us believe; rather they come *through* us. It is our responsibility to think, act and be that which we want in times of ease as well as and especially in times of dis-ease, before that which we want can 'want us.'

Where 'I.S.' the ease?

It is such a simple principle; when there is an ease within us - a *true* ease - our body and life automatically reflect this ease. Although the word ease has not yet become the new health term, the concept cannot be denied. No intelligent person today would deny that 'stress' plays a major factor in health. In addition to satisfying the physical laws of nutrition, exercise, recuperation and sanitation, (we refer you again to the Rays of the Dawn book), a truly health con-scious person would make mental and spiritual ease a top priority. By this point, there should be no question that ease is the opposite as well as the healer of dis-ease. The only question now is, where 'I.S.' this ease?

Relaxation, visualization and words of inspiration all help remind us that true healing begins with the mind. Compared with today's nor-mal practices of drugs, warning signs and focus on sickness, these positive mind techniques are a 'health' of a place to start. To com-plete the whole process of healing however, to free the ease within, we need to go further than our own mind. The Inner Self, the uni-versal source of healing, 'is' our ultimate goal. . . if we are looking for ultimate healing, that is. *Thinking* about the blissful state of ease is a mind thing, and certainly a good thing to do. But there is far more to ease and healing for that matter than meets the mind. Meditation, gradually achieving inner stillness, making the 'soul' purpose of our life to open up to and unite with our inner divine self, brings the powerfully life healing quality of ease. The

unconditional and unshakable sense of ease, (another name for
peace, faith, joy), begins when thinking turns into being, being our
innermost, highest Self. Ease, like healing, is not found, but freed.
And all human beings regardless of past imprisonments of sickness
are free to access this ease, if they have the 'mind' to do it.

Greed vs. need

The Inner Self sees no limits and neither should we. If we are to
live to our highest nature, honoring that which we are destined to
be, anything less than growing better and better each day is unnatural and unnecessary. Contrary to popular belief, it is not enough to
want 'just enough'. Asking for a little more health or a little less
pain denies the very essence of our being. We cannot believe that
we are divine beings on one hand while expecting or accepting
health problems, (as a normal part of life), on the other. Either we
are open to the unlimited energy in *anything* or we are closed to it
in *everything,* health is no exception to this rule. It takes a mind
filled with images of greater and greater levels of healing, working
with these ideas everyday to realize more of the unlimitedness of
this power.

Jesus said, "we cannot serve two masters." For our purposes here,
this can be translated to mean, "we cannot serve health and sickness." This does not mean fighting our health problems, nor does it
mean forcing health. What it does mean is allowing the healing
power to flow unresisted through us. But mentally steering the
ever moving river of physical energy into the direction of health is
our responsibility if we want to be well.

Just about the time we begin to explore the possibility that we are
heir to a greater level of healing, (and therefore happiness), than
ever imagined, old beliefs will probably surface. "I don't need that
much health." "I don't want to push my luck, if I ask for too much,
things might get worse." We have all been taught that greed is
negative. But let's not confuse *greed* with *need.* Bypassing the

laws of our nature, trying to get without using the creative process of our being and/or at the expense of our higher nature or those around us is greed. In health, wanting a pill or a person to do for us that which we will not do for our self (wanting to fix the effect without healing the cause), would be greed; it would also be futile since a health problem would continue to return until true healing is done. It is well within our right to be well as long as we work with the laws of our being. There is a great difference between *dreaming* and *scheming*.

Wanting to be well, radiantly well, is not a path of *greed*, it is one of *need*! We need to be flowing with greater and greater levels of healing in order to truly be happy and add to the happiness of others. We share ourselves and if ourselves - physical, mental and spiritual - is in pain, verbally and vibratorily, that is what we share. Does this mean we have to be radiantly well before we can help others? Obviously not, since so many who are afflicted or handicapped make tremendous contributions to the well being of others. But these are people who are working toward *their* potential for wellness. While they have limits in the physical, they choose to continue growing in the mental and spiritual. We all need to grow toward (not push for), perfection. It is our responsibility to follow the physical laws such as proper nutrition and exercise, recuperation and sanitation, as well as fill our minds with images of the health we desire, (not the sickness or pain we fear.) After that, what the power within does with our body is out of our hands. We cannot control what happens *to* us but we sure can and must create the healthiest of thoughts, beliefs and actions *through* us. And for those who in their life and health continue to lawfully reach for the top, physically and/or spiritually, the bottom never falls out.

Although we can never lose sight of the magnificence of our true Inner Self, the source of all our joy, peace and real security, ignoring the obvious pain of our false outer self, has become the occupational hazard of many spiritual and self growth proponents. The oneness of our being encompasses *all* of us; the heights of divinity to the depths of despair. If we remember the unlimited potential and power of the higher part of us, something to be meditated on daily, then revealing and healing the limited, sordid and painful part of us will be smoother. Exposing and trying to fix our guilt, hurt and inadequate feelings can put us into a deeper depression if we forget or ignore the Divine nature into which we were born. Growing and awakening to that which runs and heals the entire universe allows us to face any so called sordid part of us without fear of being swallowed up. The very nature of our being allows us to separate our Self from ourselves, our Divine nature from our so-called deficient nature. As long as we remember the true nature of our being, we can deal with the less than perfect parts of our false self without becoming stuck in the imperfection. This ability to be free from the ravages of pain and suffering, while working to heal and grow into the greater being within is a privilege sanctioned only for the human family.

The truth of a Divine power is built into all of our natures, but *awakening* to that truth remains an individual option. The choice to awaken to a greater part of us must be made from the whole of us. It is a conscious, deliberate and powerful decision that cannot be *half asked.* We grow into this higher state of being slowly and gradually. But as Jesus said, "we cannot serve two masters. . . we cannot serve God and mammon." We have to choose whether we will listen to the voice of *external getting* or that of *internal guidance.*

Missing the message because of the messenger

It is difficult to quote any bible without being accused of religious fanaticism or ideals that cannot be lived in real life. Referring to the truths of the ages always offends someone. Are we talking Old or New Testament? Is this a quote from Jesus or Moses? Truth is truth. If the message leads us to moving away from limitation and moving toward our divine unlimitedness, we must heed the message regardless of the messenger.

The wilderness of the self

Every story that has been passed down through the ages, whether fairy tale or biblical passage has two interpretations; one literal and the other symbolic. The symbolic or hidden meaning of these stories almost always contains a universal message of our higher destiny. One such story is that of Moses leading the Hebrews out of Egypt. The literal meaning is of Moses leading the people out of *physical* bondage into *physical* freedom. It took generations for this monumental feat to be accomplished and it would seem this physical release was the end of the problem, the Hebrews were free. But were they really? The Hebrews were being led to the land of "milk and honey," which they were told to "go in and possess." This should have been the beginning of paradise. Instead of the promise of milk and honey, however, the Hebrews were told by those among them that the land was filled with giants. Paradise had some major problems.

The above story was the literal, physical interpretation. There is a deeper, spiritual interpretation, not normally spoken about, one that offers a universal truth of great value to us today. Dr. Eric Butterworth explained this symbolic story in this way. He said if we look at the Hebrews as the whole human family, Egypt as the bondage of our ego or false self and Moses (the word Moses means freedom), as the freedom of our higher self, the story takes on an even greater meaning. The new land, filled with milk and honey represents the abundance that is the birthright of all human beings. The giants and other problems, 'seen' by those told to scout the land ahead of time, represents our fear and unworthiness. So what does all this mean on a universal scale? Being told of our Divine birthright to health, happiness and prosperity in all its abundance, a truth prophesied for all time, means nothing if we feel unable or unworthy to possess them. It was all there for the Hebrews *then,* as it is all here for us *now.* But if we have not fully awakened to our right to this abundance, (health being no exception), than it might as well not be there at all because it will not be there for *us*.

It is written that the Hebrews wandered in the wilderness for forty years, presumably until all the old generation of doubters and unbelievers had died out. We too can wander in the wilderness of doubt and limitation within our own self for an entire lifetime, with all the struggle, sadness and sickness that lawfully and naturally follows in its wake. But before we chalk up our suffering and problems to 'bad luck', let's see if shifting to a higher consciousness, (proclaimed by the masters of the past but virtually unlived by us in the present), can lead us to the land of "milk and honey."

Transcendence - the higher transition

"Life is getting better and better," is not just a great cliché. It is and must become the ideal upon which our life is built. This ideal of life getting better and better, (health being no exception to the rule), must be dyed into every fiber of our being. Daily and gradually we need to affirm and reconfirm our faith in such a positive ideal. This faith cannot be 'half asked.' We cannot say that our life and our health is getting better and better while still worrying that things could get worse. It is not that we must become perfectly positive in all our thinking, never to have another negative thought; that would be unnatural, not to mention impossible. But we need to have a clear direction from which the power of the universe is directed to flow. Which way do we want it directed for our life and our health? Upward and forward (better and better), or downward and backward, (worse and worse)? Unfortunately, the latter is the popular belief. Fortunately, each of us has the ability to transcend that 'B.S.'

Transcendence, rising above anything that tries to weigh us down is the ultimate goal in our quest for true wholistic healing. After all has been said and done - from visualizing the health that we want to doing all the right physical things - getting above it all is our final

choice. Lifting our consciousness to the place where dis-ease does
not exist gives that place where dis-ease *does* exist, the opening to
heal, (to whatever degree the dis-ease is able to be healed.) A
watched pot never boils and by the same token, a watched body
never heals. As said before, a conflict can never be healed at the
level of consciousness of the conflict, health problems being no exception to this rule. When we transcend - get above and beyond -
the part of us experiencing the pain or problem, we can then awak-
en to the only part of us that can heal the pain or problem. Separating ourselves from that which holds us down, allows us to connect
with the Self that can lift us, our body and our life to places that the
normal world has yet to imagine.

Of course, this transcendence stuff is simple if the thoughts that we
need to let go of had little hold on us. It's easy to transcend someone else's problem when we are not feeling what they are feeling.
What do we do, however, when the limiting dis-easing thoughts are
all we can think about? Can we really rise above attack filled anger,
gut wrenching grief or paralyzing fear?

No situation was as in need of this principle in Doreen's life as what
happened on New Year's Eve, 1996. While planning a quiet, ro-
mantic night with her husband, in one instant her world was completely turned upside down. That evening, Doreen received a
phone call that her father had had a heart attack and within two
minutes of it, he had died. A man who had sworn he would be
weight lifting until he was eighty years old, was now gone in a flash
at sixty-eight. It was such a shock and sadness, (they were extremely close), that it felt like the hole it had made would never
heal.

Doreen went through grieving over several weeks and although she
will always miss her dad's physical presence, she knew she had to
transcend the pain. They say that time heals, but if possible,
Doreen wanted to heal with little, if any, scar tissue. She knew this
meant *work*, not just time. With the grief beginning to subside, she

spent many nights asking to be lifted above and beyond this grief.
She no longer *needed* to be in pain, or feel guilty. (It seems no
matter how good we were or how much we did, guilt remains.)
She did not see any reason or any honor in denying happiness in her
life once again. Working with those thoughts, while focusing on
her present life, a peace came over her, a peace she believed would
be gone forever. Doreen had transcended to a deeper part of herself, a deeper part of all of us, and in that place, life is eternal, joyful
and secure. Rising to this place in consciousness in our Inner Self
may not change the outer conditions; sometimes conditions may reverse themselves after such a transcendence, but in this situation, it
would not be the case. Yet healing on the inside is always available, and in this case, received with tremendous gratitude.

Transcending the fine line

Once again as with all principles, a fine line exists. In transcendence, there is a fine line yet a great difference between *detachment*
and *denial*. Although we often confuse the two, the results could
not be more extreme. Detachment results in freedom and ease
while denial can only bring pain and dis-ease. Detaching from the
emotion or the situation in no way infers that neither exist; in fact,
the opposite is true. Before detaching, we must honestly admit and
unconditionally accept that which we wish to eliminate. It sounds
like a paradox but it is the heart of the principle. The situation
and/or the disturbing emotions are in our life for us to learn from;
to deny or repress their existence is to deny or repress a needed
step in our growth. Technically, we can neither deny or repress
anything, for if *we* do not acknowledge it, our *body* will.

Transcending the four most dis-easing emotions

Fear, sometimes called worry, nervousness or concern; *Anger*, sometimes called irritation, annoyance or sensitiveness; *Guilt*; sometimes called self-criticism or the should's and shouldn'ts; and *Grief*, sometimes called sorrow, sadness, loneliness or hurt, are four of the main causes of dis-ease and the main call for transcendence. These four emotions not only show a dis-ease, but a distance; the more suffering that we feel, the further we are from our home with our Inner Self. It has unfortunately become normal for these natural emotions to become unnatural. This is either due to denial or honest *un*awareness. That is why these emotions need to be broken down into more subtle terms; even the slightest annoyance is a crucial signal for transcendence.

In reality, there is no such thing as a big or deep fear, anger, guilt or grief. What seems 'big' is really years of 'little' unresolved fears, angers, guilts and griefs. In fact, when we are overtaken by a feeling - we are so angry that we could kill or so grief stricken that we could die - the wellspring of emotion, the tears that never seem to end are the result of years of holding back our feelings. It is in healing this wellspring of emotion that our true potential for wellness lies.

Does this healing of the fear, anger, guilt and grief mean that we have to dredge through our past and relive our childhood to find out if we are holding back on our feelings? Not necessarily. Every minute of everyday offers us a clue to what needs to be healed. Each time we feel nervous, irritated, should I, shouldn't I, sad or stimulated by some situation in our life, we can be sure that there is a need for healing. And if we do miss the mental signals, (worry, annoyance, etc.), we will be sure to catch the physical ones.

Wisdom is not *what* one knows, but what one *does* with what he knows. It seems that it would be of the greatest wisdom to heal our feelings, to transcend to the higher part of our Self on a moment to moment basis. It is in the slightest stir of emotion that the opening is provided for transcendence. Why wait until we are overcome with emotion to try to overcome our feeling? If we no longer need a crisis to motivate us, if we are motivated by the sheer purpose of wanting to transcend our limited self, then we will not only observe, but actually *look for* opportunities to heal. That is true wisdom.

Transcending the "old self"

"I feel like my old self again," Doreen said to Patty several years ago, following a unique experience. "That's too bad," replied Patty, "I was hoping you would have grown into a better self."

What started as a joke between Pat and Doreen in 1987 became a serious goal. They half kidded to each other that, "next year, I don't want to recognize you," but in reality, they weren't kidding. Each year, no matter how slight, their goal was to grow in consciousness, in other words, to change on the inside so that the self that they were would grow one step closer to the Self that they *really* are. Pat and Doreen had a hard time admitting, especially when one of their limitations was rearing its ugly head, but they each knew that there was an unlimited amount of work needed to be done to release their unlimited Self. They also knew that their old self, (fears, angers, guilt and grief), not to mention the health and life dis-eases that followed suit, would continue until a conscious effort was made to heal and transcend them. Pat and Doreen did not want to recognize in themselves or each other the same 'B.S.' year after year. Yet even with that focused choice, it has taken years to become somewhat unrecognizable. However, that change alone has made a world of difference in their health and their life.

Eventually, although very difficult to comprehend at the start, all we *have* been must be transcended to reveal all that we *can* be. Behind every "I am," ("I am sick." "I am lonely." "I am the kind of person who. . ."), is an *I am* we do not yet consciously know. As soon as we limit ourselves to a physical or mental "I am," we block off our spiritual *I am.* The best use of "I am" is, "I am open to learn who I *really* am."

It may be hard to imagine it now, but we need to get to the point where we transcend everything that limits or leads us away from our true divine Self. We will need to transcend our physical pleasures in life, our mental thoughts, (positive and negative), even our physical body, our health being no exception to this rule. But transcendence, as said before, means detachment, not denial. We are on this physical earth with all its pleasures and pains, to enjoy and learn from it all. Denying the physical or the mental, resisting its pleasure or its pain, refutes its very purpose. Detachment, on the other side, fully realizing while fully releasing, enjoying and/or learning, while at the same time letting go, leads us upward.

Transcendence means *awareness* without *attachment*; it means feeling what is going on within and around us without losing our Self *to* it. Step by step as we work toward listening and opening up to the guiding light within us all, the fears, angers, guilts and griefs automatically begin to heal. 'Attaching' ourselves to a path of spiritual growth instead of to how we look, what others think of us, who has one over on us and when our ship will come in, is when life becomes truly rich. Jesus probably had this ideal in mind when he said, "I come to give you life and life more abundantly." When we allow ourselves to experience what that really means, then we can see that transcending our old, limited attached "I am" self must be the way to true healing.

The eternal journey that must begin now

It really is *beyond belief.* The more that we study and experience our own healing power and watch it work in ourselves and others, the more unbelievable is the current obsession society has with sickness.

It does not take a mountain of effort or a miracle to radiate with health; health is and always has been our natural state. What does take a major effort is breaking the beliefs that block our birthright for radiant health. Old 'B.S.' die hard. It would be close to impossible to recognize these 'health' beliefs and probably impossible to heal them without taking a candid, open and sincerely honest look at our sick approach to health. Parts I and II are dedicated to that purpose. But it is up to each of us, with patience and perseverance to choose to work though our own sick beliefs toward the goal of fully functional radiant health.

After all is said and done, there is one question that remains, however. Can we afford to wait any longer before engaging in a program such as this? Of course, healing is available to all of us at any time and in any state of health or illness. We hope we have made the question of waiting until we are in pain or worse still, in panic, out of the question. What we hope we have accomplished is that we have helped provide insight and access to use valuable tools to unblock the path to wisdom. It's all in us. Letting go of the 'B.S.' that has limited us while we are in relatively good health is much easier then waiting until we are in terrible pain. This book is for those who are ready to do the work it takes to experience physical as well as spiritual radiance.

Reading **"Health beyond *Belief"*** or any book that helps us to get beyond self-imposed limitations, opens our eyes to the truth; but taking the principles, applying them in our life and actually seeing the power within work for us makes it *our* truth.

"Health beyond *Belief"* was written for a very specific purpose; to bring a forgotten radiance back to health. Getting beyond the normal barriers so we can open up to our natural abundance is for *all* areas of life. Healing our careers, relationships, even our self worth is as natural as healing the body. After years of working with friends, family, clients and especially ourselves, we have come to the conclusion that the only thing standing between us and an abundant, joyfilled life is our own limiting beliefs. The more we understand true self healing, the more it makes sense to us to get our consciousness in line with this unlimited power. As we surrender the old, ease has access to come to us. After all the stress and struggle to force life on our terms, terms that are too often sorely limited, we realize that letting go to the power that runs the entire universe brings us to a life and a health beyond what we could ever imagine, beyond belief!

****

To order more copies of Health beyond *Belief,*

Call:
908-754-5988

or Fax your order to:
908-757-5758

To be put on the Life Zones mailing list for future seminars, workshops, career opportunities and products, or to learn about how you can teach Life Zones seminars/workshops . . .

Write to:
Life Zones Services
520 W. 8th Street
Plainfield, NJ 07060

or call:
1-800-569-6900